More Time to Love

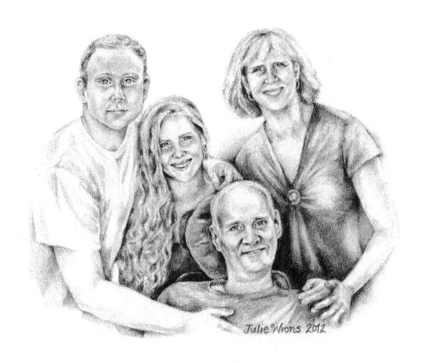

Julie Wions 2012

More Time to Love

*One Father's Extraordinary Journal
of Living Longer With ALS*

by
Joseph L. Wions

More Time to Love: *One Father's Extraordinary Journal
of Living Longer With ALS*

© Joe Wions, Dan Wions, Julie Wions

www.MoreTimetoLove.com

Drawings, hummingbird photography on section title pages,
and cover photo by Julie Wions
(See the story on p. 249)

Additional photography by friends and family members.

Your purchase of this book and art from
www.creationsbyjulie.net both support the ALS Association.

Cover and book design by Cowgirl Creative

Uplift Press
ISBN-13: 978-0-9622834-6-8
ISBN-10: 0-9622834-6-0
www.upliftpress.com

Dedication

This book is dedicated to my eternally young and
beautiful wife, Diane, and my two talented and
loving children, Dan and Julie. Their endless love
and affection have sustained me through some of the
most difficult and frightening moments of my life,
and their character and accomplishments are a
constant source of pride, inspiration, and joy.

*"The most important thing in life is
to learn how to give out love,
and to let it come in."*

— Mitch Albom,
Tuesdays with Morrie

Timeline:

2000: first symptoms
2002-2003: search for treatment begins
2003: diagnosis confirmed; first Health Update
2004: the search expands
2004-2006: alternative treatments & slowed decline
2006: an emotional turnaround
2007: spiritual healing begins
2007-2008: dietary changes & whole-being cleanses
2008-2009: spiritual healing expands & physical turnaround
2009-2010: writing the book, enjoying life
2011: golden days and misjudgements
2012 -2016: completing the work

Contents

Foreword

Joe Wions was a New Jersey college graduate having an adventure in the Rockies when he became part of my family. He lived with us for most of a year, bringing his trademark humor and warmth into our Colorado home. We kept in touch over the years as he married Diane and started wearing suits. My brothers and I were almost grownups when Joe had his two sweet redheaded kids: Dan and Julie.

My mother Louise, a community psychologist, was distressed when she heard his kids had Tourette's Syndrome, and that he had it, too. A pioneer in the self-esteem movement of the 1980s and 90s, she was distressed at new trends of pathologizing childhood, and struggled to understand the complex neurology of this disorder. When her dear friend Joe was then blindsided with his ALS diagnosis—another neurological disease—she was devastated, along with all of his family and friends.

Over the years, as Joe pursued his healing, first on a physical and then on a spiritual/emotional level, he and his family begain to unravel both pathologies and become healing experts who taught us a lot. As self-help authors, my mother and I would always envision him stepping out of his wheelchair and walking onto stages where he could move audiences in that special Joe Wions way. *Oprah would love him!*

Three years after his death, we reached out to Dan and Julie to see how we could help bring this book to life through our publishing company, Uplift Press. When we read the manuscript, we saw a side of Joe that surprised us. One of the most light-hearted people we knew in real life had become a serious writer, detailing every nuance of his powerful story. Working with Dan, who brought so much of his own self and his writing to this project, with Julie, whose art and photography enhance the book, and with videographer (and former hospice volunteer) Nick

> When Joe was living with us, I would hear gales of laughter from the kitchen. Once when I went in to see what was going on, he and my husband were making chicken. And Joe was insisting on the proper Yiddish pronunciation: "schichen." For years after that, we couldn't eat chicken without calling it "schichen," thinking of Joe and laughing at the memory.
>
> **LOUISE HART**
> LONGTIME FRIEND

Klevans, we were able to include the voices of his community—who surrounded him in life—in the sidebars to Joe's text. Dan and I also added a glossary of all the strange-sounding treatments Joe explored!

When we asked one of Joe's primary guides in his quest for healing, Dr. Wolf-Dieter Kessler, M.D. PhD. of Südbrookmerland, Germany (www.dr-kessler.net), to write a preface, Dan and I found Joe's jokester muse still hard at work with us. Kessler wrote, *"Joe Wions' extraordinary situation became the matrix to generate a man going far beyond his limits."* Kessler's profound meaning was lost somewhat in translation; and so it was with the disease. Joe was forging new territory, doubly-new since he went off the medical track to find alternative solutions that did not resonate with his known world.

Here's a 'translated' version of Kessler's touching comments:

"Despite all odds, Joe's quest for healing gave birth to a sterling life among his family and friends. In his most frightening moments he chose to care for others—his family and other ALS patients—offering a world of authentic data which can serve as an antidote against the total frustration, loneliness, meaninglessness, questioning perspective one has when lost in this disease. He became a teacher, sharing constructive evidence which he diligently collected through his own experience. Who could not admire him for that? He turned the utmost frustration into creativity. Even more, he let us share the power of love radiating from his wife, Diane, and his two children, Dan and Julie."

Kessler, who is typically successful in healing chronic disease, uses an approach called Functional Medicine (see glossary), which includes arcane but effective therapies such as Photon Therapy, Bio-Resonance, and the Quint System, which Kessler describes as "the most sophisticated, digital, and computerized method in Electro-Acupuncture available in the medical world." He remembers Joe tenderly, and wrote, "With Joe, we finally lost the battle against the non-responding neuron."

Dr. Kessler saw Joe's struggle for healing as a pursuit of innovation, and indeed, we can all be inspired by the gift of this compelling book. Kessler concludes with this inspiring thought: *"Following Joe's example, you and I are also poised to live creatively."*

—Kristen Caven, editor, March 2016

Introduction

When I turned 50, I was pretty well on track with my life plan. My wife, Diane, and I were successfully raising two extraordinarily talented children who were blossoming into caring and responsible young adults. I was earning a comfortable living doing work that I loved, and making a constructive difference in people's lives. I was enjoying an active role as a member of my congregation and was blessed with a wide circle of devoted friends and family. Life was demanding but good, and I had every reason to expect that things would get even better, and for a few years I could ignore weakness in my right leg. When a doctor told me it was the onset of ALS, I knew my good life was about to change—radically.

The odyssey that began with that diagnosis forced me to develop a new vision for my life—to rethink my sources of satisfaction, accomplishment, and happiness. I have learned a great deal about the human spirit, alternative medicine, and myself.

It sounds and feels bizarre to think of a devastating illness as a gift. Yet, surprisingly, in many ways ALS has changed my life for the better. It has been the catalyst for an unending flow of intellectual, spiritual, emotional, and even financial gifts that I never could have anticipated or imagined.

I wasn't entirely sure what motivated me to put these experiences into a book. Some of it, I'm sure, is the quest for immortality. Thinking that I was going to die, no longer "someday" but perhaps imminently, heightened my desire to leave a legacy, or, even more basically, to make a mark so as not to be forgotten.

I also wanted to leave my children more than just their memories. There was so much I wanted to share with them. There was so much accumulated "wisdom," so many moments that I expected I would miss, so many things I wanted them to know about how they make me proud, and how they contribute to the joy in my life. I needed to leave them those messages. I needed to leave them pieces of myself that they

1

hadn't yet discovered. I wanted to leave them a way to allow their children to get to know the grandpa who had missed out on them.

It was also my hope that others facing serious illness could draw something useful from my experience. Perhaps there would be lessons to be learned from my successes and my mistakes in trying to beat the odds and survive this threat to my life. It feels somewhat presumptuous to think that there might be something special enough in my own experience that it could help someone else. I am not the first person to experience nearness to death, nor will I be the last. I am sure that many have handled it with far more class and poise. It was also my hope that through sharing my feelings, others facing similar situations might feel less alone, less frightened, and perhaps be comforted by the words of another who knows firsthand what it feels like to go through something like this.

Another motivation for writing this book has been the inspiration and strength that I have drawn from the huge numbers of supporters who have donated their time and resources to help me in my quest to stabilize and regain my health. People seem to keep showing up in my life to provide whatever support I need whenever I need it. Among these people are the usual suspects: friends and relatives who have always been there for me, and I for them. But there are many others from whom I never would have expected it, who have stepped up to help out in ways I never could have imagined. I have learned to be open, accepting, and grateful about this phenomenon. It is my hope that, in sharing my story about and my learning from life with ALS, I can provide some support for others who are facing this illness, or other significant challenges in their lives. To a degree, then, this book is my attempt to "pay it forward" in return for the many gifts of support with which I have been so deeply blessed.

The book is structured in four parts. Part I, "Emerging from the Darkness," may be somewhat difficult to read, particularly for people who know me and for people who are living their own adventures with ALS. This section began as a diary of my emotions, worries, and fears. It was my way of getting things out of my system. I hope the urgency of these feelings comes through, and will provide a sense of connection and identification for others who are struggling with ALS, and understanding and compassion for those who are not.

Part II, "Searching for the Light," describes the journey of discovery on which I have embarked in pursuit of the road to recovery. This journey has included a vast amount of learning about alternative medical practices and spiritual growth. In this section of the book, I catalogue the broad array of treatments with which I have experimented, as well as the emergence of the support network that has sustained me along the way and served as the inspiration for this book. It is my hope that I will save time and money for others who are searching for ways to live with ALS.

In Part III, "Blessings, Gifts, and Insights," I describe some of the most profound lessons that I have taken from my experience with ALS and the many positive things in my life that sustain me. This section is about gratitude, appreciation, making choices, shifting beliefs, and building faith. It is my hope that this section of the book will inspire others, with or without health issues, to rethink their lives, their goals, and their capabilities in order to live healthier, more complete, more productive, and more satisfying lives.

In Part IV, "The Current Reality," I have attempted to create a picture of my current state of being and the practices that sustain me in my continuing quest for the keys to recovery. This section also describes my expectations for what lies ahead. In part, it is a call to arms for anyone who is interested in living a full, productive, healthy, and satisfying life. It is also an attempt to create a sort of roadmap to at least a partial recovery on a mental, emotional, spiritual, and perhaps even physical level.

I have been living with ALS since the year 2000. I received my confirmed diagnosis in 2003. Since the fall of 2002, I have been researching and experimenting with alternatives to traditional western medicine, which views ALS as a terminal illness with few treatment options and no hope of recovery. I believe that I am in the process of proving that it is both treatable and reversible, and I am not the only one! Sharing my experience and my conviction of recovery has now become my primary motivation for writing this book. I believe deeply in the power of the human mind, the power of will, and the power of intention. Whether you or someone you know is struggling with ALS or some other intimidating circumstance, I sincerely hope you find something in these pages that will help.

—Joseph L. Wions, January 2010

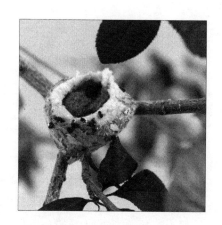

Part I:

Emerging from the Darkness

JOSEPH L. WIONS

CHAPTER ONE:

The Odyssey Begins

Like a typical golfer, I pushed on and played through the pain. It probably had a lot to do with my final shot on the sixth hole. My lie was an upward slope on the back of a knoll. I made great contact with my seven iron, hitting the ball high in the air and sending it about 130 yards. It landed gently on the upper edge of the green about 12 feet from the cup, hesitated for a moment, and began to roll. Although it was headed toward the pin, I couldn't tell from my position on the knoll if it was in line with the cup. As the ball picked up speed, I began to grow concerned that I would be facing a long and difficult uphill putt from the other end of the green. But when the ball reached the pin, instead of blowing right by, it disappeared into the cup, as if swallowed up by some unseen predator. The surge of elation that rushed through my body was so strong that I nearly came out of my shoes. It was a moment that a hacker like me typically experiences only once or twice in an 18-hole outing. It's the exhilaration of such moments that keeps one coming back to the golf course again and again, despite 100+ strokes recorded on most of the scorecards.

It was probably that shot on the sixth hole that kept me playing through the pain in my lower back and hoping for another taste of sweet triumph. I was also partly driven by reluctance to forgo an opportunity created by some unlikely circumstances. In 2000, business had mercifully summoned me from New Jersey to Florida for a few days in the dead of winter. I decided to tag on some personal time to visit my nephew, Eric. Serendipitously, my brothers-in-law, Bruce and David, were visiting from up north at the same time. This rare opportunity for the four of us to play golf together in this balmy setting in the middle of February was, well...I wasn't about to let a little back pain spoil the party.

The pain continued to build. When I got up the next morning to catch my flight back home, I couldn't straighten up. The flight was the longest of my life. Upon arrival, I was removed from the plane in a wheelchair. It took a couple of days and an epidural injection to get me standing straight again. A few days later, I cautiously resumed a normal work routine. It appeared I had dodged a bullet, and life would go on as normal.

Two months later, during our walks together, my wife noticed me dragging my right foot. When playing tennis with my son, it felt as though a lead weight was tied to it. Workouts on the cross-training machine grew more and more difficult. My energy was draining more quickly. Additional protein intake had no discernible effect. I was developing a foot-drop.

Concern over these "annoyances" led me back to the physiatrist who had administered the epidural. His EMG revealed some neuropathy. Then came the orthopedic surgeon, the neurosurgeon, more tests, and, finally, surgery. They cleaned out a stenosis (calcification build-up) in my lower back that was literally crushing the sciatic nerve going to my right leg. The surgery went well, and the doctors were pleased. I was pleased. We had found the problem and corrected it.

At least that's what we thought.

Several months later, the neuropathy was continuing to build in my right leg. It was now more than a year and a half since the trip to Florida. A brace on my right leg had become necessary to minimize the constant threat of tripping and falling. My whole leg was getting weaker. There were more doctor visits, more tests.

My neurologist, after reviewing results of several EMG studies, informed me that the neuropathy had extended into my right arm and left leg as well, even though no weakness was yet evident. He suggested I see a motor-neuron specialist in Philadelphia, suspecting something called, "multi-focal motor neuropathy," but he wanted an expert opinion. What he wasn't telling me at the time was that he feared something much worse.... Off I went to Philadelphia for one last, fairly intense, and painful EMG. Finally, after two years of wondering what was going on with my body....

I guess you can't know how you'll react when you hear the news that your life may be over. For me, it was a surreal experience. When the doctor told me what the possibilities were for a diagnosis, a wave of shock, or dread, or *something* washed over me. "Multi-focal motor neuropathy" sounded pretty tame compared to ALS. It hadn't occurred to my conscious mind until that very moment that my condition might be terminal.

The doctor was trying hard to give me something to work with, knowing I had come to him for answers about why my leg had continued to weaken, long after the back surgery was supposed to arrest or reverse the problem. He urged me not to jump to judgment, insisting that the awful options he was describing were only possibilities, and that he needed time to review all the data before he could make a definite diagnosis. Trying to satisfy my push for an answer without sending me into a panic had him navigating a very fine line.

But, hearing the possibilities, it took me a moment to absorb the reality that he was talking about *me*. It was as if I were watching a movie about someone else's experience. Following a moment that felt like suspended animation, I reacted with a surprising degree of calm.

"That's pretty much a death sentence, isn't it?"

Then the management consultant in me took over, and I shifted into data-collection mode. I had a million questions the doctor was either reluctant to or unable to answer at the moment. "It isn't conclusive," he said, trying to reassure me. There were still other diagnostics to be done and other possibilities to consider. But the most probable answer was: "Early stages of ALS."

> Joe and I were sitting on our deck when he first told me about the ominous possibilities of what he might have. All of the possible diseases were dreadful, but I prayed for any of them as an alternative to ALS.
>
> We knew something was wrong with Joe when I was 49—I remember thinking I was too young to be a widow. One of the most depressing moments was when we visited a person in Hillsborough who had ALS. After only a short time with the disease, the man was in a wheelchair and could barely move his hands. This glimpse into Joe's future was devastating. Although the visit was very informative, it left its mark on us.
>
> **DIANE WIONS**

My next appointment was a month away—the longest month of my life. It seemed cruel to make me wait that long for the definitive diagnosis, but there were others in the same position, and an earlier time just wasn't available. As my reward for enduring that wait, I learned that a definitive diagnosis still remained many months away. The tentative one was reached on June 10, 2002.

• • •

I had a long drive home from the hospital in Philadelphia where I took my first glimpse into the face of my own mortality. A crescendo of thoughts and questions swelled inside my anxious brain. My immediate concern was ensuring that my family would be covered financially. Would there be enough life insurance? Would our health insurance provide enough coverage to protect our assets? Would my long-term disability plan pay for this affliction? How long would I be able to keep working?

Several of my friends have commented that they couldn't imagine being in this position and having their first thoughts turn to financial security. Maybe it was a function of my obsessive compulsiveness, or just a way to avoid contemplating the grim realities. But the truth is, financial issues were the first things to come to mind.

Breaking the news to my family was the next of the swirling issues to come into focus. This was the most important and immediate problem for me to face, and I wasn't at all ready. I'm not sure anyone is ever ready for this discussion. As I found myself driving through parts of Philadelphia that I never knew existed, it occurred to me that I had deliberately gotten lost in order to give myself more time to think. *How do you tell the people you love so much that in all likelihood you are going to die?* I don't know what was more unbearable—the thought of having to leave them, or the sense of powerlessness to shield them from the pain this news would cause.

The pictures in my mind of what sharing the news would mean became too painful to hold on to. With my hands gripping the wheel, I shook my head and tried to re-focus my attention, but I couldn't escape the string of disparate thoughts about things that would never be. I had never bitten the bullet and paid the price to attend "Mets Dream Week" with my best friend, Lenny. Images of the Alaskan cruise Diane and I had anticipated flashed before me, along with Hawai'i and other vacations we had yet to take. The anger and overwhelming sadness of never knowing my grandchildren washed over me like a tidal wave. It sickened me to realize these things were no longer options.

This all felt so unfair! I had worked so hard to take good care of myself through diet and exercise. But I would now die younger than my father, who never kept his weight under control. How distressing that my children's future spouses would never know their father-in-law, just as my wife had been deprived of that experience with my dad.

Then, as if someone had turned on a light in a dark room, my attention shifted from inside my head to the world around me. The sky seemed brighter, the trees greener, and the need to hurry less important. I was taking keen notice of everything to appreciate life more while I still could. The old cliché about stopping to smell the roses flashed across the billboard of my mind.

I missed my exit and decided, consciously this time, to take a longer route home. I really needed to take the time to let things sink in, to adjust, to sort through all of the questions and fears and conflicting ideas that were mushrooming in my head. What would I say to my wife? What, if anything, should I tell the kids? Diane, of course, would want to know in detail what the doctor had to say. But why slam the kids with this news until I knew exactly what I was dealing with? I decided to wait on that one, as the idea brought another surge of emotion. My gut tightened. I felt my face and neck flush and my heart begin to pound. Having to look my wife and children in the eye and break this horrible news would be unbearable. I struggled to hold back the tears.

• • •

When I arrived home, I was relieved to find no other cars in the driveway. Even knowing that no one was in the house, it was difficult to get out of the car. Once inside, there would be no escape.

Anticipating the pain of the conversations that lay ahead, I wanted to run away.

It's hard to remember how long I had to suffer alone in the house with my thoughts. I was grateful that Diane arrived home well ahead of the kids. Having the time alone with her enabled me to focus on her. Little time passed before she asked me about the doctor visit. I think I was fairly successful in maintaining eye contact as I broke the news. My heart began to pound so hard that I thought it was about to burst out of my chest as I watched the tears well up in her eyes.

I don't recall exactly what we said to one another. Powerful emotions have a way of blurring the cognitive process and memory. I suspect we tried to console one another that it was only a tentative diagnosis. We would have several months ahead of us to prepare emotionally and strategically before the final verdict would be rendered.

We had many questions, few answers, and lots of decisions to make. From what we knew about ALS, time would not be on our side. The pressure was on to decide what information to pursue and what actions to take so we could be prepared without giving in to the despair of this presumed fate. For the moment, our most pressing concern was what to tell the kids. Approaching early adulthood, they would still be too wrapped up in their own lives to be acutely focused on my situation. Dan and Julie were aware that Dad had a limp, and was going to doctors to try to figure out the cause. If they had concerns about anything serious, it was not obvious at this time. I considered what I perceived as their limited consciousness of my health situation as a gift that could buy me some time. The less they asked, the less I had to reveal until it became absolutely necessary.

We decided to keep it simple. Give them only the basic information and fill in the blanks based on their request for more. This would give them the opportunity to find out as much as they were prepared to hear.

I decided to start with Dan. Even at the tender age of twenty-two, he had a pretty good head on his shoulders. As the big brother, he also had a track record of being able to help his sister through emotionally difficult situations. It seemed best to have him on board before breaking the news to Julie, who was just nineteen.

As I gazed across the kitchen table at this muscular, red-haired young man, I found it difficult to brush aside my amazement that this was the same person I had carried in a knapsack on my back just two decades ago. Then suddenly, two powerful and contrasting—though related—memories shot into my recall like a thunderbolt. I found myself flashing back to a day thirty-four years earlier, when, at the age of eighteen, I had sat by my father's side in the intensive care unit and watched helplessly as the line on the heart monitor went flat. That sense of disbelief, emptiness, and abandonment flooded back into my senses with a jolt, to be quickly replaced by the memory of a pleasant discussion I'd had with Dan on his nineteenth birthday. I had made a point of visiting him at college to make sure that he knew how glad I was to still be there for him as he surpassed the age at which I had lost my own father. "Do you know why this birthday of yours is so significant for me?" I had asked. His response caught me totally off guard and choked me up so intensely that I had to look away. He had simply said, "Yes, I know."

Now, here I sat, having to look my own son in the eye and tell him, in effect, that his time to experience that same disbelief, emptiness, and abandonment might be coming in the near future. The thought was more than I could bear. I steeled myself against my memories and shifted my focus. I wanted my attention on *his* thoughts and *his* feelings, not my own.

I began the conversation by exploring what he was aware of with regard to my dropped foot and efforts to discover its cause. Then I told him the

> Dad met me for lunch one day to talk more in depth about ALS. I remember sobbing in a food court, telling him I was horrified at the thought of losing him; telling him I was sorry for the most insignificant things...like the time I kicked a soccer ball through the garage door window, or the time he disciplined me and I vowed to beat him up when I got older. He sat across from me and focused not on his condition, but on my premature grief. Here he was, faced with the confirmed diagnosis of a disease that would turn his most prominent fears into reality...and what did he do? He parented me at the very doorway to his hell. It was way too powerful and inspiring for me to comprehend at the time.
>
> **DAN WIONS**

basics: I'd had some testing done by a specialist and had been given a list of possible diagnoses, the most likely of which was ALS. I tried reassuring him that it was early in the process and that nothing was certain at this point. Surprisingly, he had few questions. I didn't know if he was in shock or denial, or just chose to remain minimally informed for the time being. Fearful of opening doors he might not yet be prepared to walk through, I decided not to push the conversation further.

Several years later, in reflecting on this moment, Dan told me the reason for his relatively quiet absorption of the news. It turned out he knew about the path of this illness because the parents and grandparents of his friends had faced ALS. He already knew more about the disease than he cared to.

Then, it was my daughter's turn. Julie was already blossoming into a beautiful young woman. She sat where her brother had been only a few moments earlier, with her long red hair resting delicately across her shoulders. Her soft features seemed frozen in anticipation. The conversation began exactly as it had with Dan. Her reactions were equally surprising but very different. I gave her the basics and asked what questions she might have. My expectation had been that she would prefer to remain as oblivious as possible to the harsh reality. Instead, she generated an endless stream of questions. She wanted to know what ALS was, how quickly it would progress, what the impact would be on me physically, how long I would have to live. She went on and on, inquiring with a startling passion, as if searching for the right question or the right number of questions that would somehow make the nightmare disappear.

It's hard to remember any conversations in my life that have been

> When Dad was first diagnosed, it was the scariest thing I had ever come to face. Not only was I losing a loved one, but, as a teenager still learning to cope with my own illnesses, I was also losing a safety net and life guide during a time when I needed it the most. Above all, I feared the struggle and tragic suffering that lay ahead for my father. His insight, guidance, and humor often helped give me perspective in the moment. Dad consistently made it clear that, while being thrown into this deep dark ocean of unknowns, we would somehow get through it together, and we would all learn how to swim. And we did just that.
>
> **JULIE WIONS**

more difficult to face. I felt a peculiar kind of strength as I focused on my children's reactions. The conversation was about the possible end of my life. Yet, all I could think about was how they were handling it and what I could do to minimize the impact on them. Discussing the possibility of my impending death as if it were some sort of a book report was like an out of body experience. At the same time, it was a tremendous release. Despite the threat that lay ahead of us, at least now we were prepared to face it together as a family.

One family member who was spared all of this was my mother. Prior to the date of my final diagnosis, the ravages of dementia had already taken a cruel toll on her. There was no point in troubling her more. My stepfather, George, was not so lucky. Even now, more than six years after my diagnosis, despite my efforts to focus on the bright side, I can hear the anguish in his voice when we speak on the phone.

On May 6, 2003, approximately eleven months after my tentative diagnosis, Mom passed without ever knowing the cause of the weakness in my leg. Three days later, with Diane by my side, I returned to Philadelphia to hear the doctor confirm that the cause of the weakness in my leg was, in fact, ALS.

CHAPTER TWO:

A Future Denied

Having lost my father at such a young age, I had been forced to grow up prematurely. I had been responsible and accountable for myself for a long time. When I became a management consultant, I made my living by teaching and coaching people in the art of intentional and assertive living. I considered myself a fairly strong person who could face adversity, make adjustments, and move forward. But facing my own mortality presented me with a new kind of challenge. During that first month, after learning that ALS was the most likely explanation for my lame right leg, I found myself lost in the depths of despair, struggling not to drown in a deep pool of frightening thoughts and emotions.

It was impossible not to anticipate what it would be like to live out one of my worst fears: paralysis. I had already struggled with the ravages of another neurological condition, Tourette's Syndrome, since I was a boy. While I had become quite adept over the years at masking my symptoms, the urge to twitch—to relieve the tension in my shoulders, wrist, neck, ankle, stomach, or scalp by squeezing my muscles in just precisely the right way to erase the discomfort—was sometimes overpowering. And this obsessive need to flex the muscles in the perfect way would sometimes compel me to writhe for hours trying to hit the mark, leaving me exhausted, frustrated, and in considerable pain. I had developed an ability to refocus my attention in order to limit and avoid this unfortunate scenario with considerable, but not complete, success. As if paralysis were not enough to deal with, what was I going to do with that powerful urge to twitch if I couldn't move? It was hard enough trying to keep my sanity now, but if I couldn't move, and the urge kept pressing, then what? The thought was horrifying!

I also struggled with the idea of a tracheostomy and needing a feeding tube to go on living, and the possibility of a tortuous death by slow suffocation as my diaphragm wasted away, which is how ALS often ends. And, after spending most of my adult life earning my living with my ability to articulate and influence others with words, how would I cope if I lost my ability to speak? I was also an active and athletic guy. What would I do for recreation without tennis and skiing and hiking? Hardest of all, the thought of not being able to hold my wife or my children in my arms reduced me to tears.

But my worst fear was not of death or disability. It was the fear of leaving my family without sufficient resources. That was what drove me most in those early days of coping with the diagnosis. My days filled up with managing monetary issues—planning housing scenarios, trying to figure out how to leave my family with a foundation that would ensure a roof over their heads, food on the table and a reasonable shot at a normal life after I was gone. What scared the hell out of me was the thought of them suffocating under a mountain of debt born of accessibility modifications to our home, mounting medical expenses, and in-home care when I was no longer able to function on my own. The discomfort, the immobility, the physical helplessness would be hard enough, but not knowing if my wife and kids would be secure was unbearable.

Throughout my life, even as a child, I had been meticulously organized. I knew what I had, and I thought I knew what I needed to do with my money. But the idea of making a mistake that I might not be around to correct took me well out of my comfort zone. I spent hours on the computer constructing one what-if scenario after another, trying to figure out the best alternatives for managing our available assets. This was the kind of situation when it was good to have a friend with the right skills, especially one who was as close as a brother.

Lenny and I have been best friends since our sophomore year in college. He and his wife, Mona, and Diane and I all met within the same year. The four of us have been as close as family for almost forty years. We have done everything together. We got married a year apart, bought our first homes a year apart, started our families about a year apart, vacationed together, celebrated our own and our children's achievements together, and comforted each other over the loss of loved ones.

Through the years, as our careers progressed, we also used our playful, sibling-like sarcasm to keep each other's egos from getting overly inflated. I remember helping Lenny "wordsmith" his essays for grants and applications through law school and beyond, never missing an opportunity to comment on how such a bright and successful guy could be so incredibly illiterate. It would certainly be appropriate for me to claim the lion's share of the credit for the enormous strength of the well-exercised middle finger on my best friend's right hand. Today, the name Leonard J. Witman is one of the most respected in the field of U.S. tax and pension law. The minute he heard about my diagnosis, he was there to help sort out the finances and help us plan for the contingencies.

It would be several years before I became fully cognizant of just how much fear was driving my behavior in those first few months. Yet fear was not the only heavy emotion that was clouding my life. Movies, commercials, and scenes from everyday life were having a profoundly different effect on me. Scenes of weddings would get me emotional about not being there to walk my own children down the aisle. Scenes of small children at play would trigger thoughts of the grandchildren I might never know. I found myself daydreaming about sharing words of wisdom with my kids when they would come to face the trials of parenthood: the one time in a parent's life when a child is finally ready for advice, and I might not be around to give it! I had always pictured myself and my wife, aged but trim and vibrant. We would be walking in the woods or

> Joe was a very meticulous and systematic man, even when we first met him as a freshman in college. It became our ritual that I would go into his dorm room and rearrange his hairbrush. Every time Joe came back to his room—for four years—he would begrudgingly return it to its original spot, rolling his eyes each time.
>
> This act symbolized our lifelong friendship of over forty years, not just as the closest of friends but also like brothers who would lovingly tease one another. Whether traveling with our families, watching sporting events, or annual holiday traditions, you would always find us laughing.
>
> **LENNY WITMAN**
> BEST FRIEND FROM COLLEGE

rocking on a swing beside each other as the two of us watched an orange sun melt slowly and gracefully into the western sky as it kissed another day good-bye. These were all visions of a future denied.

There were so many things I wanted to be there to say, so much wisdom I wanted to share. I was plagued with worries of how to leave notes behind and have them available at the time they would be needed. What I wanted to say to my son and daughter was:

Please tell your children about me. Let them know who I was, what I was like – and make sure to put in some of the nice stuff! Tell them stories about Grandpa. Tell them about our trips to baseball games, about playing catch and soccer and Frisbee in the backyard. Tell them about our vacations in Florida and Vermont, and our trips to Disney World. Tell them about my playfulness, my silliness, my teasing, and how hard I worked at trying to be there for you when things got difficult. Tell them how much I would have loved them, and how much I wish I could be there to hold them and play with them. Remember me to them.

• • •

Life in the early months with ALS was a dichotomy of extreme emotions. On the one hand, I was preparing to die, and, on the other, I was fighting to continue living. I recorded notes on my computer in a sort of diary, unable to figure out what else to do with the overwhelming flood of intense emotions from my melodramatic struggle.

My chest and gut tighten, my eyes fill with tears, and I fight the urge to give in to feeling sorry for myself. It feels so unjust. I have tried so hard to be a good person. I have dedicated my life to helping others. I have sacrificed so much for my children. Why, why am I being denied the privilege of

> Even with his declining health, Dad still found humor in playfully chasing me around the driveway in his motorized wheelchair. His mind and his sense of humor remained sharp while he made the best out of the situation.
>
> **JULIE WIONS**
>
> Some of the fondest memories I have with my dad were of the two of us driving in the car listening to Billy Joel's greatest hits. He would often sing along....I would often tell him he was out of tune...He would then often sing louder and more out of tune.
>
> **DAN WIONS**

seeing them build their own families? Why am I having the golden years with my beloved stolen away so close to my grasp? We live in quest of purpose and answers. It is hard to find purpose in this affliction. There seem to be no answers.

Yet, it is what it is. My only choice is how I will deal with it. If my time is limited I refuse to live it as a victim. Why would I choose to spend such a precious resource in such a frivolous and unpleasant way? If I have limited time, let me squeeze every ounce of living out of it that I can. Let me create as much as I can. Let me work feverishly to leave this world in better shape than it was when I entered it – in whatever ways I can touch it with the time I have left. There is no point in wallowing. It produces nothing but more pain. It changes nothing except for leaving me with less time to live. What a waste it would be.

Yet, the temptation looms incessantly. It would be so easy to give in to the tears. And what would be so wrong with shedding a few tears? If nothing else, it could provide some release. The trick is to sense when the release is enough and to shift my focus back to action, or back to appreciation of the beauty I still have time to enjoy.

Sometimes, while sitting in the shower trying to gather the energy to dry myself, I linger too long and think too much about the growing physical constraints imposed by this disease. Soon, I find myself fighting off the sorrow, the frustration, and the anger that my arms and hands just won't work the way they used to. Then comes the fear that one day soon my arms won't work at all. The emotions quickly become overwhelming.

Friends and relatives often ask me how I cope with the daunting threats and realities of having ALS, and the toll it takes on the body and mind. As I sit in the swirl of these emotional storms, those early questions and my responses come back to me again and again. *If my remaining time here is limited, why would I want to squander it by playing the victim?* Whenever these words echo in my mind, I realize I am behaving in discord with my intention, and this mantra always seems to jar me loose from the grasp of the pain. Around this time, someone shared with me the words of a dying man whom he greatly respected: "Pain in life is inevitable...suffering is optional." So, after a moment or two of emotional release, I learned to command the storm to leave, dry myself off, and get on with my day. I learned I don't have the luxury of time to suffer.

Wrestling with the notion of a "terminal" diagnosis was a surreal experience. I often felt more like an observer than participant. I guess that came from the disbelief … a sense of, "This can't be happening to me." Things like this are what you read about in the papers or hear about on the news. They happen to other people. But thinking that this could be the end of *my life* threw me into an interesting paradox. I knew full well that my mental state and attitude would have tremendous influence on how my illness would progress. Remaining positive, hopeful, and determined to survive—while simultaneously preparing for the end of my life—seemed a very bizarre juxtaposition of perspectives.

I set to work dealing with concrete tasks. For instance, we had bills to transition to automatic payments, and tons of files and papers to purge and reorganize in ways that made sense to Diane. I didn't want to leave her with the burden of years of accumulated paperwork: financial records, health records, old client files, and more. And she was delighted to see increasing amounts of available space in our file cabinets. I was often unsuccessful in resisting the overpowering temptation to procrastinate, but my compulsiveness drove me to comb through each individual file—to be sure I was not going to discard anything that might be needed after I was gone. But it was not compulsiveness alone that entrapped me in this level of detail. With each file, I found myself confronted with a decision about who might need the information in the future, a future in which I would likely no longer be a part. Throwing away a file felt like discarding a piece of my life and my history. It was as if there were an unspoken assumption that, as the files disappeared, so would I. Regardless, I would have to learn how to relinquish control so that someone else could take over when I was no longer able.

As the atrophy brought on by the disease ate away at my muscles, I began to melt down to a significantly smaller person. My waist and shirt sizes kept shrinking, and I gradually had to replace much of my clothing. Buying replacements wasn't too difficult. My wardrobe needs were much simpler once I stopped working. Letting go of clothing that I was fond of was much more difficult. Giving it away kept bringing home the realization that I was literally disappearing from the planet.

Along with the atrophy came a parade of aches, pains, and weaknesses. Most difficult to handle was the thought that the motor-neuron specialists put in my head that this illness is a one-way street. In other words, when you lose strength in some part of your body, it's gone forever. On the other hand, the impact of fatigue, worrying, and physical or emotional stress can cause a temporary loss of ability. For a while, for example, my hand could dependably write a check one day and then not the next. And the day came when I couldn't do it at all. Changes could occur over hours or even minutes. Some mornings, for instance, I could hold my electric toothbrush well enough to get the job done non-stop, and some mornings I would have to take several breathers. The problem with ALS and other motor-neuron diseases is that, every time strength diminishes or a pain emerges, you can't tell for a while whether it is just temporarily due to fatigue or stress, or whether it is progression of the disease. It can be very challenging to resist panic.

Being declared terminally ill presents an amazing paradox to managing your perspective. On the one hand, you want to remain positive and optimistic, since it is fairly well established that our emotions affect our health and that a positive outlook can help promote healing. Plus, it just makes more sense to enjoy your limited time than to squander it in self-pity and worry. Yet, while you are trying to maintain that positive outlook and enjoy what is left of the gift of your life, you have to prepare for the end. To do otherwise would amount to living your final days in denial and behaving irresponsibly toward those whom you must leave behind.

CHAPTER THREE:

Considering the Alternatives

It takes a while to get past the surrealism, to *really get it* that how you are spending your time right now is how you are choosing to spend what is left of your life. When this idea finally sank in, I had to make a choice about what I wanted to do. What statement was I going to make with the rest of my life? What was I going to produce? What model was I going to set for my children about how to handle this level of adversity? How did I want to be remembered? It finally hit me that holding on to my normal patterns wasn't going to do anything but burn me out and cause me to fade away with no additional contribution to myself or anyone else. It was time to face the fact that my life had changed dramatically. *I either needed to redefine myself or let the illness do it for me.*

Once I *got it* that things had to change, I began to shift my priorities. My work was no longer being a management consultant. My work now was to demonstrate how to take responsibility for my own survival and live with the intention to find a way to beat what many call an unbeatable disease.

The most pressing issue at the time seemed to be resolving our living situation. Our home of nearly twenty years was very dear to us. We lived in a wonderful community with lots of friends, surrounded by a fairly rural environment with lots of wildlife. We did not want to move, but the house had too many steps, some narrow doorways, and other constraints that would become increasingly difficult for me to negotiate as my mobility declined. The imposing costs of renovations, in the face of the huge medical expenses we were anticipating, forced us to consider making a move.

On the other hand, this house was pretty much the only home my children had ever known. Dan and Julie were toddlers when we moved in. Diane and I loved the house, the property, and our incredible network of friends and supporters. The psychological and emotional impact of leaving our home while simultaneously trying to adjust to the probability of my impending demise was more than a bit overwhelming. Complicating the process even further was the very real possibility that I might be gone before my mobility limitations became an issue. I needed to stop the ambivalence. I had to get this decision off my plate so I could focus on other things.

This is where my friend, Jim Bunce, jumped into the picture. Jim and I had been friends since college. Over the years, we had shared a good deal of social and recreational time that was so filled with laughter it took on an almost therapeutic quality. Jim is a very large and very strong man with an almost cherubic face. His delightfully twisted sense of humor somehow finds the lighter side of almost anything that happens from moment to moment. A mutual friend of ours once compared Jim's sensibilities to those of the late Sam Kinison: loud, boisterous, and outrageous. Yet, by contrast, Jim always seems to deliver his mockery of the human condition without ever being offensive or obnoxious. At a time that I was wrestling with the notion of my own mortality, Jim's company was just what the doctor ordered.

We were both at an age when we were interested in looking into retirement communities. My medical condition had given me some added incentive to explore this possibility. Jim had suggested that we spend some time together investigating some of the newer communities that were mushrooming in our area. Designed with people over fifty in mind, they seemed like logical alternatives to renovating my existing home. After visiting a few developments, though, my decision became clear. Designs of the new homes, the constraints placed on modifications by the builders, and the costs of the homes eliminated most of the financial advantages of a move. Factoring in the emotional trauma of leaving a home that we loved brought me to the obvious conclusion. We would renovate and stay put.

• • •

While I realized that my days of working as a management consultant were numbered, it took me about a year to refocus my energies primarily on healing. When my odyssey began, I knew very little about alternative medicine. But when a doctor looks you in the eye and tells you that you have a disease that comes with a one-way ticket to the cemetery, it leaves you with two choices: you either accept the doctor's pronouncement as inevitable, or you turn to paradigms beyond the traditional medical model that offer alternative viewpoints and possibilities. I chose the latter.

A few weeks after my initial diagnosis, I was presented with the opportunity, at a quarterly business meeting, to inform my friends and colleagues at my firm of the doctor's findings that I probably had ALS—a disease that was eventually going to kill me, leaving me paralyzed and physically dependent on others along the way. During a break in the meeting, a good friend and colleague, approached me and asked, "Would you consider something outside the box?" I looked him in the eye and said, "I've just been given a death sentence, and the conventional doctors have nothing to offer me but how to cope with dying. What have I got to lose? I'll look at anything."

That was the beginning of my adventures into the world of alternative medicine. I was introduced to Dr. Kessler, the first of many alternative practitioners who have contributed to my efforts to halt the

> Toward the end of high school, I watched the grandfather of one friend, and the father of another, wither away to ALS. Both men followed the traditional medical paradigm, hoping for the "Hail Mary" of a miracle cure, as they died a little more each day. While I respected their decisions, and felt compassion for their conditions, I watched my Dad choose a path that had no clear direction; a path on which he had to figure out the rules for himself.
>
> When I was young, the first nightmare I ever had was about a giant gorilla chasing me. In the dream, Dad showed up out of nowhere and kicked the gorilla's ass... like REALLY kicked its ass. The gorilla was crying and everything.
>
> My dad had been my hero since I was a kid. But when he made the choice to take his life into his own hands, I saw him for the first time as being courageous.
>
> **DAN WIONS**

progression of my illness, reverse my symptoms, and regain my health. This began my adventure, and my ongoing challenge of determining which practitioners and practices were worthy of my time and limited resources. After this moment, I began focusing my attention on discovering new paradigms and procedures that offered me the possibility of restoring my health.

. . .

Dealing with things like housing, medical treatments, and the dreaded finances were only the tip of the iceberg. The real challenges weren't so much about what was on my mind as they were about the way my mind was working. One of the most basic issues I found myself confronting was my mind-set regarding living vs. dying. This led me to adopt the following philosophy:

Death is an event. It happens once in a lifetime. Living is what you do until that event stops you from doing it. Even with a "terminal" illness, I believe that I still have a choice. I can focus on the dying, or I can focus on the living.

It seemed to me that many people with terminal illnesses tend to focus on dying until it finally happens. It also seemed to me that, by focusing on the dying, these people actually invite and hasten the process. I believed this to be a terrible waste of the final chapter of one's life, which can also be the defining period of one's life, a time to display some character, make a statement, and choose how you want to be remembered. I decided I wanted people who know and care about me to remember me for how I lived and what I had contributed to the world, not for how I died. I chose (and choose every day) to focus on living until the end, rather than focusing on dying until I accomplish it.

In a phone conversation with my friend and colleague, Thom Radice, I remember him commenting on what he viewed as an absence of any evidence in my behavior of feeling sorry for myself or playing the victim. While I clearly have moments when I struggle not to go there, I have consciously committed myself to rejecting what I consider such dark and irresponsible behavior. It was flattering and validating to hear in my friend's words that, at least to him, I was achieving some degree of success in avoiding self-pity. As I said to Thom, "If my days are numbered, why on Earth would I choose to spend them feeling like that!?" *Why would I want to waste the precious time I have left doing anything less than living my life as fully, productively, and enjoyably as I can?*

Instead of suffering, I chose to search for meaning in this misfortune. Maybe I got this disease because God needed someone stubborn enough to refuse to die from it—someone determined enough to find a way to beat it. If I were to be successful in doing that, think about the contribution it would make to others with the affliction. Even if I were to dedicate myself to this effort and fail, the worst case would be that I set an example for my children on how to face adversity with dignity and determination, and provide my family and friends with memories they could reflect on fondly rather than with pain and grief.

> Dad showed me how to create a world in which I can be limitless; a world where "no" is not an option. He showed me how to adapt in order to thrive. I thank him for instilling in me the values and tools that have enabled me to grow into the woman I am today.
>
> **JULIE WIONS**

Admittedly, all of this sounds very cerebral. The emotional experience, on the other hand, has posed a constant challenge to my mind's ability to stay in "living" mode vs. "dying" mode. Every day I have to remind myself of the choice I made to find a way to defeat what doctors call, "an always-terminal illness." Every time my breathing becomes more labored or my arm becomes more difficult to move, it tests my resolve to live up to that decision, and to believe in the possibility of my success.

• • •

Another aspect of my mind-set that had to shift was how I defined what it meant to be a man. I had always been a fairly active guy. My weekly routine included three to five trips to the gym for resistance training and cardiovascular work. During the warmer months, I jogged five to ten miles a week. Recreationally, I enjoyed tennis, skiing, golf, backpacking, hiking, and softball. I was always pretty handy and enjoyed playing "Mr. Fix-It" around the house. Yard work—trimming and planting shrubs and trees or vegetable gardening—was like a mini-vacation. I really enjoyed being outside. Not only did I engage in a wide variety of outdoor physical activities, I was also pretty good at most of them. Golf was the most glaring exception, but I just enjoyed the hell out of it.

Planning and organizing were other aspects of my life that played a significant role in defining who I was. I took care of the finances, making sure that the bills were paid, investments were growing, and money was available when big expenses hit unexpectedly. I planned all our trips, whether for business, vacations, or exploring colleges. If an automobile or an appliance needed to be replaced, I was the one who did the research and negotiating. Diane and I had always been a good fit, partly because I was the one who obsessed over the big picture, while she kept us busy in the here-and-now. We shared the big decisions and bringing in the money, but I was the one to keep an eye on how things fit together and how each part affected the whole. I was driven by the notion of taking care of my family. For me, this was a much larger part of being a man than the macho stuff that took place in the gym or on the playing field.

> Throughout our marriage, Joe was the person who took care of things around the house. Although our "job descriptions" changed when he could no longer perform certain tasks, I always felt that he still took care of us by his presence and inner strength.
>
> **DIANE WIONS**

When you start to have trouble pulling on socks, tying shoelaces, buttoning buttons, pulling up zippers, handling utensils, or stirring a pot of vegetables, however—well, it's hard to feel virile. Dan took over routine chores like putting out the trash and recycling and bringing in firewood. Julie started doing more for me around the house as well. Diane, with a demanding teaching job that required long hours, had to take over most of the bill-paying when I could no longer hold a pen to write a check. Watching the increasing pressure on my family as my physical capabilities diminished, it became harder and harder to feel like something other than a burden.

Noticing how much of my manhood was tied to my physical self was quite a revelation. Perhaps I had overestimated just how evolved I was as a person. Recognizing and accepting that I had to evolve much further on this idea was not easy, but it was critical. My failure to accept this reality amounted to an all-expenses-paid trip to victim-land and severe depression. *I had to relearn what it meant to be a man without the use of my arms and legs.*

Slowly the insights began to emerge. My brain was still fully functional; my problem-solving capabilities were undiminished. Even without my muscles, I could still be there for my kids and my wife when they were feeling overwhelmed or uncertain about how to proceed with a difficult decision. I could still take care of some of the bill paying and record keeping with the use of the computer, the phone, and credit cards. And the strength it took to remain positive and productive in the face of adversity gave me plenty of opportunity to demonstrate my manhood.

Making this mental transition was helpful, but my new reality kept me humble. When difficult problem-solving conversations with a spouse, child, or friend were interrupted by my unavoidable requests to scratch the itch on my nose, move my foot to eliminate a pressure pain, or bring a urinal so I could take a pee—well, they had a way of making me feel a little less powerful. And so this thought process was a slow and difficult evolution.

• • •

ALS is a cruel adversary, and it doesn't progress the same way for everyone. In my case, it started as a foot drop, and then a gradual weakening of the right leg. Next, it began to affect my hands and fingers, my back and hip flexor muscles, then my shoulders and arms, my left leg and foot, and ultimately my breathing. It took about four years from the onset of symptoms for the disease to make a significant impact on my breathing. The more symptoms progressed, the more noticeable small changes in function became. Sometimes, changes occurred slowly and seemingly deliberately. Writing, for example, grew increasingly difficult, but at a very slow pace. At first, my hand would tire quickly. Then, it would be difficult to hold it steady. After that, it became almost impossible to hold a pencil, let alone move one across a page.

Other losses would occur more suddenly. As my legs weakened, I needed increasing amounts of assistance to get around. At first, I used canes, then walkers, then wheelchairs. One day I could drive, the next day I could not—I got in the car and realized I could no longer raise my foot quickly enough to use the brakes safely. Only a couple of blocks from home, I turned around and came back, knowing that my driving days were over. Another time, after a trip, I returned home to discover I could no longer climb the six steps to my kitchen from the den.

As physical ability erodes, the disease robs you of independence, and inflates the time required to complete basic functions. When 60 to 70 percent of your waking hours are consumed with things like shaving, showering, dressing, eating, physical therapy, and taking medication or supplements, it becomes increasingly difficult to accomplish much in a day. The cruelty of the disease doesn't end with the erosion of physical abilities and your sense of independence. It also erodes your ability to take care of your family and feel productive.

Staying positive in the face of such circumstances requires conscious and focused effort. Every day you are blasted with evidence that you are dying. As you gasp for air, exhausted from the effort of typing an e-mail or washing your hands, you count your blessings and accomplishments to remind yourself of the loving family and army of caring friends that are there to support you. You recount the people you have helped and the things you have achieved in life, and you try to let go of the goals that may not be met. You enjoy the sunshine and value the rain for the green it will produce.

• • •

One final shift in perspective that I had to confront was how I cared for myself. For most of my adult life, I had followed what I thought was a fairly healthy lifestyle. My father's ruptured aorta had taught me the importance of diet and exercise, and I wanted to spare my children the trauma I had experienced. I was living confidently, under the impression that I was doing all the right things to avoid his fate. And I was right. But ALS had taught me was that I was ignoring a critical piece of the puzzle. I needed to learn how to "oil my nerves."

People who take good care of their cars know how important it is to change the oil regularly. They know that a well-oiled machine runs better, has fewer problems, and lasts longer. I have always been one of those people, and I have gotten great performance and longevity out of my vehicles. I would never abuse a car by waiting too long to replace a part or grease the joints or change the oil.

Yet, I have spent a lifetime justifying abusive behavior to my own body by convincing myself that it was necessary to do so in order to keep my commitments to others. I would stay up way too late, crunching out one more e-mail. I would grind out one more bill or one more computer-file update or one more design for a client, all in the names of responsibility and accountability. I figured that, since I ate well and exercised regularly, I could handle the stress. Instead of listening to my body when my self-imposed pressures were causing it to scream for mercy, to take a break, to do something fun for myself, I would continue to grind it out.

Sure, I took vacations, spent time with my family, hiked, gardened, skied, played tennis, and spent valued time with friends. What I never learned to do, however, was truly relax. I spent too many years walking around with my neck and face muscles in a knot. I didn't take enough time to meditate, to listen to the birds sing and the wind blow through the trees, to deliberately do nothing—to oil my nerves. I always had to be doing "something."

After years of enduring this self-imposed and unrelieved stress and the accompanying over-production of adrenaline that kept me going, I believe that my abused body responded with an autoimmune dysfunction that began to attack my nervous system. When you abuse any machinery, it will eventually break down. In my case, this break-down took the form of ALS. I'd be interested in a study that explored a link between ALS and certain personality types, as I have known many hard-driving and intense people who have gotten this disease.

My new question was: "What do I do about it now?" Was it too late to learn how to oil my nerves regularly? Even though doing so may have amounted to something akin to a personality transformation, I couldn't see that I had much choice. The best the motor-neuron specialists could offer me was a meager attempt to slow the inevitable, with no hope of recovery. I had nothing to lose, and everything to gain, so I let the learning begin.

My brother and I had severe cases of Tourette's Syndrome, the symptoms of which were often triggered by our father's voice. At times, being in the same room for more than ten minutes could be unbearably painful. Eventually, as he worsened, it became clear to us that we somehow needed to learn to conquer our lifelong disorders, to be there for him. The change he modeled for us, along with his patience, support, love and strength, catapulted us into an intense journey of self-awareness and growth.

JULIE WIONS

CHAPTER FOUR

Biting My Tongue

So much happened in the eleven months between the tentative and the confirmed diagnoses that the news seemed almost anticlimactic. When the final verdict rolled off the doctor's lips, my gut contracted in response to the verbal blow, but quickly released. I had already explored the depths of despair. I had already begun preparing for the worst case. My emotions had already run the gamut in anticipation of this moment. There was a sense of finality, a sense of, "Okay, it's real," but I had already addressed the question of, "What am I going to do about it?" I had already placed the western medical paradigm in its box and had begun to search for other models that offered hope of conquering my horrible adversary.

Months before this news came, I had made my first visit to the Kessler Clinic in Germany. I was already on a regimen of homeopathic and herbal supplements designed to address the toxicities that were impeding my body from healing itself. Not yet fully prepared to abandon traditional medicine, I had hoped that I would be able to persuade my neurologist to collaborate with Dr. Kessler to enhance my chances of success. I had printed out some materials from Kessler's website to introduce the neurologist to his work, but the doctor completely ignored the papers in my extended hand and went on talking about his findings. This unmitigated display of arrogance was so offensive that it took every ounce of emotional strength I could muster to bite my tongue and hold back my opinion of his behavior. Across the small examination room, I could sense Diane poised to intervene, fearing that I was about to display the more aggressive side of my personality. But I successfully suppressed my urge to tell him off, not wanting to would alienate the key person that I needed to

convince my insurance company of the legitimacy of my disability
claim. We would be desperately dependent on that income once I
decided to stop working and focus on fighting my illness. I decided to
put my feelings aside and simply observe the doctor's pathetic display
of ego.

As we were preparing to leave, I had one last question for the
doctor, though. Having never experienced such extreme circumstances,
I had no idea what the requirements would be to convince the
insurance company that I was disabled enough to collect on my policy.
I asked the doctor, "How bad off do I have to be before the insurance
company will agree to pay?" His response was somewhat reassuring,
but again displayed the degree to which he was so thoroughly
impressed with himself. He said, "You tell me when you want to stop
working and I will make it happen. I have never lost a case."

What I didn't know at that moment was that the confirmed
diagnosis of ALS provided me with a slam-dunk case to execute my
disability insurance. The doctor would have had to be a low-grade
moron or simply intent on screwing it up to prevent the activation of
my coverage. It's probably all for the best that I lacked this knowledge
at the time. The result would not have been one of my more shining
moments, and I am sure that Diane would have let me know it.

• • •

Diane had very little to say during our session with the doctor.
She sat quietly and took copious notes on the doctor's conclusions and
his answers to our questions about how things were likely to progress.
On the way home in the car, the reality of what we had heard began to
weigh heavily on us. Having dealt with a good deal of the emotional
trauma over the previous eleven months, my mind became immersed in
contingency plans. All of the anticipated issues—finances, housing,
treatment options, and use of time—now demanded concrete decisions
and actions.

Absorbed in these thoughts for a while, I became painfully aware
of the quiet stillness to my right. I glanced over to Diane, noticing her
bowed head and feeling the somberness of her mood. She has never

been quick to share her concerns. Diane is one of those people who is always first to shine the light of attention on others. She is adept at showing interest and drawing out from other people what is going on in their lives, but when *she* suffers, she tends to withdraw and struggle with her demons in solitude, which is hard for me to witness. Determining when to give her space and when to intervene has long been one of the most difficult things for me to manage in our relationship.

Acting out of my own inability to tolerate her distress, I decided to break the ice. As delicately as I could, in a half-whispering tone, I asked, "What are you thinking, Di?" Her response gripped my heart like a vise. "I don't want you to die." She choked out the words, fighting back tears with mixed success. We were standing on the threshold of a level of pain that was threatening to sweep us away. There was nothing we could do about the hand we had been dealt. The only choice we had available was how we would deal with it. I have no idea where I found the strength or perspective to shift the mood, but, in response to her desperate admission, I blurted out, "Too late!"

The air cracked with the burst of laughter that exploded from both of us. As I reached out and took her hand, the loving energy that flowed between us eased the moment. There was a sense of reassurance that whatever time we had left together, we could still choose to enjoy it.

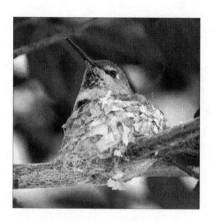

Part II:

Searching
for the Light

CHAPTER FIVE:

An Early Retirement

Some people look forward to leaving work behind, but I loved what I did. I had managed to define what my life was about, lay out a game plan, and follow it. My work with Guttman Development Strategies (GDS) represented the fulfillment of a career goal. Prior to joining the group in 1992, I had spent more than fourteen years preparing myself for work as an external management consultant. I was living my dream, doing the work of my choice with people for whom I had great professional respect and with whom relationships were mutually supportive to a degree most people only dream about. I hated being forced into an early retirement. Howard Guttman had created a unique business structure, bringing together highly skilled professionals working as peers, and minimizing the corporate politics that derail good working relationships. The result was the most talented and collaborative group of people with whom I was ever privileged to be associated.

For more than ten years, I had worked effectively and proudly as part of this group, coaching executives, building effective teams, and teaching management skills. By the time of my conclusive diagnosis, in May of 2003, however, the typical practice of carting my carry-on luggage and briefcase around city streets on business trips was beginning to feel like an Olympic-level competition. The weakness in my leg would frequently force me to stop and rest before I could cover a city block.

At this point I had been wearing a custom-fitted leg brace to support my right foot for more than two years. This device counteracted the foot-drop and reduced the risk of tripping and falling, yet it had enough give to allow my foot to flex and exercise to avoid more rapid atrophy. The brace made it possible for me to walk with a little more confidence and speed, but sadly, it couldn't stop the muscle fatigue.

One night, on my way back from a job in Indiana, a mix-up at the airport caused me to miss my flight from South Bend. I jumped back into a rental car and raced to Chicago's O'Hare Airport to catch the last available flight back home to New Jersey that night. When I got to O'Hare ten minutes before my scheduled departure, the rental car attendant generously offered to shuttle me all the way to the terminal, driving me with abandon and dropping me off with minutes to spare. But as I raced down the concourse, dragging my bags behind me, I could feel the strength draining from my right leg. Out of nowhere, a room filled with wheelchairs appeared to my right. With my departure time only two minutes away, I poked my head in the door and explained my dilemma to the airport employee. He popped me into a wheelchair and raced me down the concourse, delivering me to the gate just as the flight attendant was preparing to close the door.

But I could not rely on rooms full of wheelchairs appearing every time I got tired. It was apparent that it was time to make the big choice. I could continue to work until the end, leaving my family with a pile of loose ends, or I could stop now and devote myself to getting things in order, focusing my energies on the search for a way to beat this disease. Even if the disease won, at least there would be time to do something about securing my family's future. Diane and I had several daunting decisions to make: How far could we stretch the insurance and how would it be used? What renovations would we make to the house, and who would do them? What medical equipment would we need, and where would we get it?

I'll never forget the day I had to look my colleagues in the eye and tell them that the diagnosis was conclusive. I had to tell them that I would be backing away from work to take care of myself and my family—engaging in a battle I neither sought nor wanted—in order to survive.

It was June 2003. We had just completed our quarterly business meeting, and Howard had told the group that I wanted a few minutes to speak to them. Seventeen faces stared back at me across the long conference table in anxious anticipation—all of them hoping not to hear what they feared was coming. I struggled to hold back the tears. Several painfully long minutes passed before I could muster my composure. After a few long, deep breaths, I choked out, "This is even harder than I thought it was going to be." There was no easy way to say it, and I couldn't bear to torture them, or myself, by drawing things out, so I simply told them that, during my recent visit with the neurologist, the diagnosis had been confirmed. "I have ALS."

As I fought to maintain eye contact, I was overwhelmed with the ambivalence of feeling both immensely supported and increasingly pained by what I saw in their eyes. For more than a decade, we had shared challenges and triumphs and had come to know each other on very personal levels. It was evident from the looks on their faces, the misty eyes and the choked voices, that this message was as difficult for them to hear as it was for me to deliver. The pain in the room was palpable. Shoulders and heads drooped like leaves falling off trees in an autumn breeze. Some fought back tears. Others sat in stunned silence. It was impossible to bear the collective pain for very long.

I went on to share my painful decision to pull back from work, prepare for the unwanted changes that lay ahead, and intensify my search for alternative ways to stop the disease progression and reverse its symptoms. Gisele wiped away a tear and promised her ongoing support. Robert caught me completely off guard with the acknowledgment, "This is what courage looks like." Others took their turns with words of encouragement and pledges of support. As time would reveal, their pledges were far from empty.

Over the years, as my condition progressed, the strength of the bonds I shared with these people became even more evident. Many pitched in with substantial financial support and made the effort to stay in contact, despite their incredibly demanding schedules. A few of them made extraordinary efforts, both to support me directly and to help me find resources.

My friend Klaus Oebel and his wife, Carol Bocchino, the one who introduced me to Dr. Kessler, went out of their way to provide information about contacts and resources there to ensure that my first visit would go as smoothly as possible. They shared a great many of their personal experiences with Kessler's clinic to ensure that I was well-prepared for that initial visit. Over the two-and-a-half years that I was to be under Kessler's care, they made it a point to stay current with my experience and the results from my visits to Germany. They were always ready to provide perspective, insight, and support regarding any issues that arose along the way.

> The first time Joe and I worked together, it was at his home. He made lunch for me and when the plate arrived, on it was a smiley face–cherry tomato eyes, cucumber nose and a red pepper mouth in a big smile. It brought a huge grin to my face and every time I smiled at him, I told him it was *my* 'smiley face.'
>
> **JUNE HALPER**
> COLLEAGUE AND FRIEND

Other members of the group also found ways to pitch in over the next few years. My friend June Halper became a regular contributor of weekend help to provide some relief for my live-in health aides. Barbara Weber and her husband, Jim Kenny, although not members of my congregation, were quick to jump in when my synagogue arranged a rotation of people to provide meals on a monthly basis. In addition, Barbara has worked to channel financial support from the group as a whole.

Each morning, when I get out of bed and look out my window to the backyard, I am greeted by one of the most enduring symbols of my colleagues' ongoing support. About a year after my formal departure from the group, my declining mobility led us to build a ground floor, wheelchair-accessible bedroom. Led by Barbara and our colleague, Dona Lee Calabrese, the group rallied to the call of a "garden party" to landscape around the addition. They pooled their resources to purchase and deliver shrubs, topsoil, and mulch. On the day of the "party," over twenty people showed up, including consultants, administrators, office workers, spouses, and children, to dig, cart, and plant for about five hours. They even brought food and took care of the clean-up. When they were done, we had a beautiful array of foliage and flowers surrounding the outside walls of our new bedroom. Some of these people traveled for more than two hours to participate in this event, and did so with an unforgettable level of enthusiasm, playfulness, and dedication. I still proudly wear the t-shirt, bearing a picture of all those present that was created to commemorate the event.

Every summer, GDS holds a family picnic to celebrate its successes, give its members a chance to get to know each other's families, and have some fun together. Years after my departure from work, my colleagues not only continued to welcome me and my family to these events, they treated me almost like a celebrity when I arrived. They'd line up to greet me and spend personal time catching up on events and finding out how I'm doing. In 2004, a year after my retirement, I arrived at the picnic still walking, with the help of canes. By 2005, I needed a motorized scooter to get around.

In 2006, I made quite a dramatic entrance. Extremely excited about seeing my former colleagues, especially since I wasn't getting out of the house much at that time, I had rolled my power wheelchair into our wheelchair-accessible minivan. When Diane turned the key in the ignition, a loud "pop" announced the death of the air conditioner compressor. My spirits sank like a brick in water as we quickly realized the oppressive heat of this July day would prohibit our use of the vehicle. I was crushed.

Unable to bear the thought of missing the picnic, I snapped out of my funk, called the dealership and was able to negotiate the swap of their last wheelchair-accessible rental for my vehicle so they could repair the air conditioner while we proceeded to the picnic. We arrived about an hour late. I was exhausted and overwhelmed with emotion. My friends rushed to the car to greet me. I felt at once like a conquering hero for simply having arrived, and a revered loved one for the display of attention exhibited by the crowd around my car. As I struggled to find the strength to extract myself and my wheelchair from the car, I remember Howard expressing his amazement at my tenacity with the words, "What a warrior!" It was only at that moment, hearing Howard's flattering description of my behavior, that I realized how hard I had worked to get there and how important it was for me to have come.

As of this writing, it has been more than six years since I was forced by circumstances to end my work relationship with these people. They are far more than colleagues to me. I continue to feel deeply touched and awed by their continued support and unwavering interest in my wellbeing.

CHAPTER SIX:

A World of Possibilities

The Search for Treatment Begins

In the year before my confirmed diagnosis, our search for effective treatment began when my colleague introduced me to Dr. Kessler's "outside the box" practice.

Dr. Wolf-Dieter Kessler introduced me to what he called "Functional Medicine," a whole new paradigm for healing the human body. His treatment ranged from dietary changes, homeopathic remedies, and lots and lots of dietary supplements—including learning how to inject myself with vitamin B12—neuro-biofeedback, sound therapy and other forms of frequency testing and treatment, chelation, work on my immune system, and so on and soforth.

From October 2002 through January 2005, I traveled to Germany six times for Dr. Kessler's treatment. I found myself fascinated with his practice. Through Functional Medicine, he seeks to eliminate toxins and strengthen the body's functions in order to unlock its self-healing powers. This is far different from the pharmacological and surgical treatment of symptoms that dominates western medical practice. But, as I eventually learned, this focus on unlocking the natural self-healing mechanisms is a common feature of all alternative modalities. What makes Kessler's approach unique is the breadth and depth of it. The vast array of methods and machines, coupled with his traditional and alternative medical training, gave him a powerful arsenal to address my ALS. He had an extraordinary capacity for identifying and prioritizing the key issues to address in fighting a chronic illness. His tools included muscle-strength testing, electro-dermal testing, chelation, blood oxygenation, foot reflexology, frequency testing and treatment, homeopathy, and a variety of other methods of diagnosis and treatment, most of which I had never encountered before.

Along with the doctor's impressive track record in treating chronic illness and a personal style that blended warmth and humor with stereotypical German rigidity, I found this almost-mystical menagerie of methods irresistible, and let myself be whisked away into a brave new world of possibilities. Kessler never made any promises of recovery, but the confidence he expressed that he could slow down the progression of my disease was new and exciting and hopeful and such a far cry from the death sentence I had received from my American doctors.

In addition to the medical treatment, my excursions to Germany included a significant social element. The people at the clinic were warm and friendly; each visit felt more and more like a reunion with friends. In particular, I became very attached to my hosts, the Samuels, whom I stayed with during five of my six visits. Anton and Gerda Samuel consistently went out of their way to accommodate me. During my earlier visits, I would rent their spare apartment upstairs and share some meals with them and their children, Andre and Inka. By the final visit, they were rearranging furniture to accommodate me in their own living quarters, building ramps to ensure my wheelchair access, and treating me as a houseguest.

As I prepared to take professional leave from work and wage war with ALS, I promised my colleagues at GDS that I would keep them informed of my progress. The mechanism for doing this became a periodic e-mail called the "Health Update." It started out as a short progress report on changes in my physical capacity, emotional status, descriptions and results of treatments, news about my family, and the boundless gratitude I felt for the ongoing support of those receiving the e-mail. As time went on, friends and other supporters outside of my work group learned about the "Health Updates" and would often ask to be included in the distribution. The list quickly grew to a hundred names or more. I have been averaging about four of these e-mails per year for several years now. Here is the first health update, which I wrote shortly after my third visit to Germany. Diane accompanied me on this trip.

HEALTH UPDATE: 7/13/03

Hi Folks,

Just wanted to let you know we got back safe and sound from Germany, and to update you on my progress. There are so many of you who have expressed interest in how I am doing that I figured the easiest way to keep everyone up to date is to send out an occasional e-mail. So, here is the first edition.

I went through my regular treatment with Dr. Kessler in Germany the week before last. It appears that my body is making some progress in resolving the issues that are blocking the self-healing process. My gluten and lactose intolerances are under control, but I still have to be careful.

In addition to the regular treatment, Kessler also put me on a continued program of chelation therapy to remove metals from my system, using both oral form and injections, which I will continue at home.

I am also equipped to begin use of the VIT Organ treatment, using a serum comprised of my blood and a protein extracted from sheep cells. This therapy has been documented to have the potential to halt the progression and even to regenerate muscle mass. Next week, I will begin the use of neuro-biofeedback, a third therapy that could halt the progression. So, there is a lot of hope, but no results to report as yet.

While in Germany, I was able to be much more
mobile than I expected. We did a lot of bike
riding and walking. It was exhausting but
encouraging to be able to move around on my own as
much as I did. I am still, however, experiencing
significant weakness in my right leg and left
hand, although there have been no significant
lasting changes to report in the last couple of
months.

Hope you are all doing well.

Joe

It was quite a treat having Diane join me on my second trip to
Germany. She got a chance to meet all of the people who were taking
such good care of me at the Kessler Clinic. She also came to
understand why I was falling in love with the Samuels. Gerda and
Anton were two of the warmest and friendliest people I had ever met.
They had welcomed me, and now Diane, into their home with open
arms and endless hospitality.

When Diane found out that their little girl was taking piano
lessons, the music teacher in her emerged with a passion. Diane was
teaching middle school choir at that time and Inka Samuel fell into that
age group. She insisted on hearing Inka play and proceeded to
playfully and lovingly coach her through an informal lesson.

At the end of the week of our treatment at the Kessler Clinic, and
our stay with the Samuels, Diane warned young Inka that she would be
back, so she had better practice her piano. Inka giggled at Diane's
playful threat. We shared our parting hugs with our hosts and left for
the airport.

Since Diane was accompanying me on this trip, we decided to
extend our stay by a few days and do some sightseeing. Doctor
Kessler's assistant, Karen, escorted us to the train station to make sure

we got off safely on our short vacation. Our destination was Berlin. This was an unusual choice for us. Our vacations were more likely to include national parks than major cities. My friend, Klaus, who was quite familiar with the city, had suggested Berlin, and by the end of our four days there I was quite grateful for his guidance.

As a Jew, visiting what was once the seat of power for the Third Reich was both a startling and a moving experience. We visited buildings and bunkers that once housed the Nazi elite and still bore the bullet holes and bomb damage that had been deliberately left unrepaired as reminders to the German people of a dreadful path once taken. One of my most vivid memories of Berlin's painful past was a bombed-out church partly held together by huge bands of steel. We were told by our tour guide that the structure had been deliberately left standing for the power of its message. The dark, eerie, almost ghostlike structure surrounded by the modern architecture of a new era seemed to scream out the words, "Never again!"

Beyond the heavy history lesson, there was also quite a bit of beauty to enjoy in the city. Louise Hart, a longtime friend who lives in California, had serendipitously planned a visit that coincided with ours. One day, we rented bicycles and rode from West to East Berlin, taking in as much of what the city had to offer as we could cram into a day. We enjoyed the floral beauty of the Tiergarten (Berlin's version of New York City's Central Park); rode through the Brandenburg Gate; and visited art museums, cathedrals, and synagogues.

While the bicycle enabled me to see a lot more than would have been possible using only my canes, the extensive pedaling was beginning to take its toll by late afternoon. Traveling up a slightly inclined street, it occurred to me that I

> Joe lived with my family in Boulder when he was a young man seeing the world. We always had fun playing together. Over the years, whenever we saw each other, memories of previous fun times would kick off new ones. When we rode bikes in Berlin, we remembered horseback riding in Colorado. At a trot, he had started yelping, and so had I. He made jokes about "loads not properly strapped down." We laughed and yelped even louder! Joe's sense of humor helped him handle all of life's indignities, which multiplied exponentially with ALS.
>
> **LOUISE HART**
> LONGTIME FRIEND

might have gotten too far ahead of Diane and Louise. As I reached out for the curb with my right foot, my knee buckled and I slowly tumbled to the ground. It felt as if I were falling in slow motion. A mixture of embarrassment and relief overcame me as I settled onto the pavement. Cars passing by stopped to see if I was all right and my companions rushed to my aid. Aside from the embarrassment, I was unharmed. It seemed that ALS was determined to remind me that there were limits to my enjoyment of the day.

Unwilling to yield to the pesky disease, I took a few minutes to rest, climbed back on the bike, and rode on. We crossed back into West Berlin, returned the bikes, and found a quiet little bistro for dinner. Following a wonderful meal celebrating my birthday, Diane and I said our goodbyes to Louise and enjoyed a leisurely evening walk back to our hotel. While pleasant, the walk was not short. We stopped several times to give my weary right leg a chance to recharge before reaching our destination.

During the time I was seeing Kessler, I had also found practitioners closer to home offering treatments with the potential to supplement, and perhaps enhance, the results I was getting in Germany. These treatments included neuro-biofeedback, chelation with intravenous EDTA, and sound therapy. Using sound therapy and chelation, I was able to make significant strides in reducing the heavy metals in my body. In particular, these approaches helped to significantly reduce the mercury that had accumulated in my cells over the years. Still, there was no reversal of muscular weakness. In the following health update, I refer to: the neuro-biofeedback and sound therapy treatments, which I received from Dr. Rima Laibow in New York; chelation therapy, which I received from both Dr. Kessler in Germany and Dr. David Strasserberg here in New Jersey; and to some other treatments in Dr. Kessler's program.

HEALTH UPDATE: 8/29/03

Well, it's been about a month and there have been no dramatic changes. I was hoping that by now I would be able to tell you I was signing up for dancing lessons, but I guess I'll have to put that off for at least one more update. The best news at this point is that there seems to be no significant progression of the ALS. There is some increased weakness in my left hand, but it is not consistent, and it is difficult to tell whether it represents progression of the disease or just a reaction to some of the treatment.

I am engaged with Dr. Kessler's "Vit Organ Treatment," which involves a series of injections, drops, capsules, and pills that will take me into October or November to complete. Diane and I also completed the neuro-biofeedback training. As soon as we figure out how to make the software work at home, we will begin implementing the procedure about three times per week for about six weeks. I am also continuing to use sound therapy to try to reduce some of the toxicity that contributes to the ALS.

Chelation is a process that removes metals from tissues. We discovered that my mercury levels are off the charts, and there is a strong connection between mercury and ALS. Although it can be done orally and/or intravenously, the oral program has been making me ill. So, we are working hard on how to get it out. One positive note is that we recently retested for the metals after four weeks of sound therapy, and discovered slightly lowered mercury levels. Consequently, we are continuing with this therapy a while longer.

We are continuing to uncover issues that have contributed to the ALS, and are trying to address them with these therapies as they become clear. It's a pretty comprehensive attack, and we need a

little more time to see results. I remain pretty
hopeful, if for no other reason than that the
alternative really stinks!

Hope you are all doing well.

                                    Joe

No one in the conventional medical world or in alternative
therapy guarantees to halt the progress or reverse the symptoms of
ALS. The difference is that alternative practitioners evoke the hope
that, if you can get the body functioning properly, you can overcome
any illness—even ALS.

The problem is that many of these therapies are extremely
expensive and not reimbursable through insurance. Moreover, some
practitioners are all too eager to take your money with little evidence
that they can actually make a difference. I was fortunate to have the
personal resources and the additional financial support from friends
and family to pursue quite a few different options. At least three of my
trips to Germany were financed in part by frequent-flyer miles donated
by friends.

Even with this kind of help, I spent tens of thousands of dollars
trying to find therapies that might make a difference. Over time, I
learned where to invest in reasonable possibilities and how to avoid the
money pits. It was an expensive education. Many people battling this
disease cannot afford to do what I have done. This was part of my
motivation for writing this book: to help others avoid the expense of
my lessons. In Chapter 21, I will elaborate on what has worked best.

HEALTH UPDATE: 10/22/03

I was hoping to report dramatic progress in
reversing symptoms by now. Unfortunately, I'm not
there yet. The good news is that I am still
standing, walking, driving, preparing my own
meals, and generally performing the basic

functions of daily living. But it is quite a bit more challenging than it used to be. Ah, the things we take for granted.

Depending on how much sleep I have gotten or how much I have pushed myself, my energy level can vary from day to day. Last night, I should have gotten to bed earlier, so my body feels a little heavy today, and walking is a little more laborious than usual. My left hand continues to weaken at a very slow pace. I can still use it to do most things, but I'm not the guy you would want to ask to hold onto an expensive piece of China.

The neuro-biofeedback and sound therapy seem to be going quite well. While there has been no noticeable physical response, my brain patterns are showing progress on the computer, and the voice analyses show continued progress in reducing mercury, pesticides and other toxicity levels.

The stem cells and the Vit Organ Treatments hopefully are doing their work, but similarly have shown no overt signs of regeneration of nerve or muscle tissue. Both of these treatments began in July, and I am told that they can each take six months to a year to have impact, so there is still time for them to help. While the stem cells were a one-shot (literally) deal, the Vit Organ Treatment continues. I am still administering pills and/or injections on a daily basis and will continue with this for a number of months yet. Although there is no clear evidence in my physical condition that any of these treatments have helped, I also have to consider that progression of the ALS might have been significantly more pronounced by now if I had not been doing all of this. In a recent visit to my motor-neuron specialist, he told me that even though many ALS patients experience significant declines in that period of time, he sees no significant progression of the disease over the three months between visits. This is encouraging.

The latest addition to the arsenal is a new protocol of supplements from another doctor in Germany who has been doing some cutting-edge research in auto-immune issues. Dr. Kessler recommended another doctor, Dr. Flavine-Koenig, thinking that her work offers a significant additional weapon in the fight against ALS. I began taking the new regimen of pills today. These supplements are designed to reverse a process that creates intracellular toxicity, which contributes to the destruction of nerve cells. At least, that is my best understanding on how to describe it in plain English.

I have also made some progress in dealing with the chelation issue. Basically, I have switched from using EDTA IVs to taking DMSA in pill form. BioMark, a company in Atlanta that produces and administers stem cells, claims to have experienced better results chelating ALS patients using DMSA without the side effects I was experiencing from EDTA. I just started using the DMSA this week, and so far so good. Hopefully, this will resolve a major obstacle in my detoxification to date.

Well, that's about all I have for now, and hopefully not more than you needed to know. Thanks again for your continued interest and support.

Joe

I tried sound therapy as well. I spoke into a microphone hooked up to a laptop and watched as the soundwaves were charted. Each coordinate on the chart was assigned to a given toxin from a vast database—everything from household chemicals and pesticides to heavy metals. They drew my blood to double-check the voice analysis. Bert, the tech, turned to me and asked, with a grin, "So, how long ago did you fill up your gas tank?" Bert had found Hexane (a chemical compound found in refined petroleum and crude oil) on my sound chart. I was floored—I had filled it up on the way there.

Bert explained to me that every known piece of matter on the planet has a resonance point, or frequency at which it resonates most intensely. As a musician, this made a lot of sense to me. I could recall countless practice sessions in rooms where one or two notes on my instrument would resonate far beyond the sound other notes I produced. His software program had compiled the resonance points of every known toxin in its database. Medically speaking, I learned that, often, when a toxic substance finds its home in our body for an extended period of time, many of our immune system's warning mechanisms move on to more pressing issues. Our body will chemically alter itself to accommodate our environment.

Once my analysis was finished, I watched Bert program a medieval predecessor of the iPod with ten different audio tracks. Each track contained the resonance points of the ten most urgent toxins I needed to address. Bert then put a pulse oximeter on my finger and played each track to test me. He explained that the frequency and its inverse would both work to bring my immune system's attention to the dormant toxin in my body, but my body would respond favorably to one, and not the other. On each of the tracks, one frequency would raise my oxygen count while lowering my pulse, and the other would have the opposite effect. Surprisingly, we wouldn't have actually needed the pulse oximeter at all. For whichever frequency my body rejected, I began twitching (a common symptom of Tourette's) almost uncontrollably. The opposite frequency would relax my body immediately. The realization that this stress was caused by mere sound exposure was fascinating to me. I wasn't having any type of obsessive compulsive reaction to the sound. My body was merely physical and unconscious. It shed light on one of the potential reasons why certain types of music had always done more to relax my body and alleviate my Tourette's symptoms than pharmaceutical drugs.

My treatment plan was to listen to the ten tracks once a day. Each session would take an hour, and I was welcome to do other things while I listened. I followed this sound regimen for two weeks. When I went back for my next appointment, I saw a print out of my blood tests confirming the accuracy of the sound therapy diagnostics from my first visit. Another round of testing showed that my Mesozoic MP3 box had reduced my ten toxin levels by 60 to 100%. Over the course of many months, we were able to determine which toxins had been dormant for a while and which were only recent exposures. This allowed us to also determine how much of the elimination process was attributed to the catalyst of the sound therapy vs. my immune system's ability to merely do what it was designed to do, without any external aid. The results, especially with heavy metals, were impressive.

DAN WIONS

Throughout my adventures with ALS, I have met many people who were also engaged in dealing with this illness. Some of them have tried some of the same things that I have tried. Others have experimented with different therapies. Still others have stayed with conventional medicine. Through the exchange of information, I have learned a great deal about assessing which therapies might be worth pursuing. It has helped me to make increasingly better and more confident decisions about where and when to apply my resources. The fear of missing the "best" opportunity for effective treatment and the constant pressure of being in a high-stakes race against time don't provide the best context for good judgment. Through my personal experience and conversations with others in my situation, I have learned to ask more and better questions before writing a check for a new treatment. Yet, since research data on alternative modalities is scarce, personal experience and gut feelings continued to play a large role in my selection and/or continuation of treatment modalities.

HEALTH UPDATE: 12/19/03

Well, another two months have passed since my last update, and the best news I have to report is that I am still standing, driving, working out, preparing my own meals, and generally performing the basic functions of daily living independently. Walking, however, continues to grow more challenging, as does the use of my hands, especially the left one. While I can still push around and lift a surprising amount of weight at the gym, fine-motor tasks can be unbelievably challenging. Buttons and zippers continue to be antagonists for me, but with patience and perseverance I can usually overcome their tenacity. The good news is that they don't seem to be much more challenging than they were two months ago.

A couple of weeks ago I got fitted for two new braces. I got to try them on for the first time today. One is a replacement for the one I have been wearing on my right leg for the past two years to keep my foot from dropping, so I don't trip and fall. The new one gives me a lot more support and makes walking much easier. I am looking forward to breaking it in and using it more frequently, although I have to be careful not to overuse it. Since it restricts my ankle movement more, it could allow those muscles to atrophy faster. The other brace pulls my shoulders up to keep me from hunching over due to weakening and shortening of the hip flexor muscles. I won't have that one for a couple of weeks yet, and will have to be careful not to overuse it, as well, to avoid more muscle atrophy.

On the treatment front, there have been a few minor changes and adjustments. I have elected to stop the neuro-biofeedback, at least for the time being. It has removed a significant amount of muscle tension from my head, neck, and shoulders, but I am not convinced it is going to do very much for the ALS, directly. And the cost is becoming quite a burden.

The sound therapy, combined with the switch to DMSA, has been remarkably effective in detoxifying my system. It has eliminated a number of pesticides, metals and other toxins, and significantly reduced my mercury level. We still have some work to do on mercury and lead and a few other things. So, the sound therapy will continue until we are successful in "getting the lead out!" (Sorry, I couldn't resist!) ☺

The stem cells, hopefully, are having some effect, and the Vit Organ Treatments continue. While there is yet no clear result from either of these, I won't be able to assess their impact with any certainty until a full year has passed. That will be next summer.

Since beginning the protocol of supplements to fight intracellular toxicity, my condition seems to have stabilized to a degree. It is very difficult to tell if the progression has stopped, but it seems to have slowed even further. However, the changes are so subtle that it is hard to know if they are real. We have added injections of B12 and folic acid to the protocol. At first, I was doing this daily; now it is weekly. This may be the approach that has had the biggest impact since my initial treatments with Dr. Kessler. He continues to be a strong ally, and we are in frequent contact by phone and e-mail. I will be going back to Germany the first week in February for more treatment at his clinic.

We are currently looking at another potential treatment that I would have to go to the Bahamas to have administered initially. (I know, it's a dirty job, but someone has to do it!) It involves oral sprays and daily injections of something called peptides. The formal research on it is somewhat questionable, but they claim to be compiling impressive empirical evidence that it helps slow progression, and in some cases ALS patients have regained recently lost muscle function. They have been using it with MS patients for a longer time and have recently started using it with ALS. I have some serious questions about

the efficacy of this treatment, but if I get
convincing feedback from those who have tried it,
it may be something I'll explore further. I will
need to be convinced that there is a highly
probable payoff, since the cost is about $10,000 a
year, not counting the expense of traveling to the
Bahamas every three months to pick up more
supplies.

Well, that's about all for now, and hopefully not
more than you needed to know. Have a wonderful
holiday—whichever one you celebrate—and a Happy
New Year!

Thanks again for your continued interest and
support.

                                    Joe

    Getting to and from Kessler's clinic was quite a routine. I would
typically board a flight in Newark around six o'clock in the evening
and arrive at Frankfurt about seven thirty the next morning. Then,
barely conscious, I would board a commuter flight to the town of
Bremen in the northwestern part of the country. From there, a car
would pick me up for the hour-and-a-half drive to the tiny hamlet of
Victorbur, the home of the clinic.
    On the return trip from my third visit, in July of 2003, ALS once
again reminded me why I was engaging in these long journeys. Bremen
has a nice but fairly small airport. In contrast to the enclosed, carpeted
tunnels that are characteristic of jetways in larger airports, the ones in
Bremen consist of rubber-mat-coated metal ramps encased in a plastic
tube. The day of my departure, it had been raining, and there was some
moisture on the walkway. Halfway down the ramp, my left foot went
out from under me, and my weakened right leg collapsed in the blink
of an eye. I found myself sitting on my left foot with my "good" leg in
considerable pain. There I was, four thousand miles from home,

terrified by the thought that I might have broken something and wondering how I was going to get back.

The airline attendants quickly rushed to my aid and helped me to my feet. As my leg straightened out, I realized that the pain was coming from my hyper-flexed knee. After a few minutes, the pain subsided to a tolerable level and I was able to walk on very carefully without assistance, board the plane, and head home.

ALS has a very twisted sense of humor.

CHAPTER SEVEN:

Exotic Machines

and Stinky Chinese Herbs

Between my fourth and fifth visits to Germany (February and July
2004), I had incorporated two new modalities into my treatment plan.
One was an herbal remedy developed in China that had shown notable
promise for the reversal of ALS symptoms. It had been brought to my
attention by my friend Ralph Russo, who had also been recently
diagnosed. This concoction, called BNG, would arrive packed in large
zip-locked bags, about ten or twelve to a carton. In its uncooked state,
the contents of one of these bags looked like something collected by a
six-year-old off the forest floor. It contained leaves and twigs and
berries from various plants and even a dose of leech dust. A lengthy
double-boiling and filtering process resulted in five days' worth of a
dark brown tea, plus a special stench that pervaded my entire house for
hours. That nose-holding fragrance was the subject of frequent
commentary from friends and family who had to endure it.

The other modality that I added to my regimen was acupuncture.
Twice a week, for five months from August through December 2004,
Dr. Fen Xie adorned my body with needles in the hope of channeling
healing energy to my decimated nerves and muscles. The following
health updates catalogue the ups and downs of my experiences while
using BNG, acupuncture, and continuing to see Dr. Kessler
simultaneously. I also explored a few other modalities along the way.

HEALTH UPDATE· 2/27/04

January was a scary month. The progression
appeared to be accelerating, and the motor-neuron
specialist confirmed in late January that I had

lost some strength in my arms, legs, and hands. I didn't really need him to tell me that, but harsh reality confirmed that I was not imagining it.

The changes have not been dramatic, although they can be humbling. My fine-motor skills have gotten a little worse, and I have grown more sensitive to fatigue and cold. There are times when using a knife and fork is a challenge. I can do it, but sometimes I drop a utensil or find myself having to grip my fork or spoon in my fist instead of the normal finger grip. The pinky on my right hand tends to wander away from the ring finger, and is sometimes difficult to control. Typing is still quite doable, but I have to sometimes get creative to reach a "p" or an "a" on the keyboard.

Walking and staying upright have become much harder as my core muscle strength weakens, especially when I have to use both hands to do something, like washing a dish. Using both hands to wash a dish keeps me from bracing myself on the counter. This puts considerable strain on my neck and back to keep me vertical. A friend recently provided me with a walker that has wheels and a basket. It makes it a lot easier to do things like bring in the mail—an extraordinary feat when both hands are occupied by canes.

Getting out of bed in the morning has also become much more difficult. My body requires a lot of sleep now, and is considerably weakened throughout the day if I don't get it. Stretching exercises in the morning make getting up an even lengthier process, but help to maintain my range of motion and avoid pain.

On the plus side, the progression seems to have stabilized somewhat again. I am still able to walk short distances, drive, and prepare my own meals. I continue to be optimistic that there is some way to beat this thing, and am grateful that the rate of progression is remaining slow enough to give me the time to search for the solution.

On the therapy front, there have been a number of changes. I spent the first week of February back in Germany getting my system reassessed. We have made significant progress with detoxification, but there is still some work to do. Dr. Kessler decided that we have given the Vit Organ treatment enough of a test, so we have discontinued it. Which is too bad—I was actually beginning to enjoy those three or four jabs in my gut every week. (Not!) We also identified progress in strengthening some internal organs and systems to improve my overall metabolism. I returned home with about two-dozen new homeopathic remedies to dissolve under my tongue to address the most pressing current issues. Ironically, I may be aborting those and many of the other substances I have been taking as I venture into a new treatment called Bu Nao Gao (I know—you just can't make this stuff up).

> Over the years, Joe and I met for lunch every so often, as he worked for other pharmaceutical companies and eventually became a consultant. Joe was always even-tempered, even as he met many challenges that would have sent others over the wall. He has always impressed me with his incredible optimism, drive, curiosity, ability to see all sides of issues, and creativity in working out solutions and pathways forward. I am inspired now by his ability to adapt, survive and thrive - in his loving family, as a professional, a role model and a friend.
>
> **ANDREA ZINTZ**
> FORMER COLLEAGUE

Bu Nao Gao (or BNG, as I will refer to it from here on) is a Chinese herbal brew that has been used in limited clinical trials in China with ALS and some related disorders with amazing success. There is a private, worldwide trial going on right now with about 75 patients that is being overseen by the developer of the concoction, who still lives and works in China.

Both he and his physician-daughter are highly reputable neurologists. The daughter's practice in the U.S. is focused on ALS and other neurological diseases. They have had success in 80 to 90 percent of the cases in achieving near or complete stabilization of the disease. This is exciting stuff, even if it does have a funny sounding name to the non-Chinese ear. It requires brewing some herbs into a tea-like concoction that I have to pour down my gullet twice a day. I will be starting on it in about a week.

I was very close to going to the Bahamas for the peptide treatment, when a friend and fellow ALS patient introduced me to the BNG. While the peptides have shown some interesting results as well, reports from users are not as impressive. The peptides will restore energy and balance, slow progression, and return some recently lost function. These are no small gains, but my concern is that I have not heard from anyone that they "stop" progression. I have only heard they "slow" progression. BNG, on the other hand, holds a more consistent promise of stopping progression and restoring lost function on a more permanent basis, with a possible retreatment after a few years. The peptides, on the other hand, require constant use to retain whatever gains you get. Oh well, no fun in the sun for me.

I have suspended the sound therapy for now, but the jury is still out on whether I will pick it up again. I am currently doing some additional testing for a more accurate read on the level of heavy metals in my body. This will help me determine whether or not to resume the process. The health food stores keep getting wealthier from my focus on organic produce, which helps avoid exposure to other kinds of toxins.

We are under contract for the accessibility renovations on the house. Now, all I have to do is figure out how to pay for it. We have enough equity in the house, but now is not the time that I want to be increasing our debt.

If my body doesn't start to regain some strength soon, I'm going to be looking into getting a motorized scooter to help me get around outside. That will save a lot of energy, but will incur yet another expense. I am now on Medicare, so the insurance gets a little trickier. If I spend the insurance money on a scooter now and wind up needing an electric wheelchair later on, it may be more difficult to get Medicare to cover it, and the wheelchair will cost about ten times what the scooter will. The assistance fund set up by our synagogue has been helping out big time with some of these expenses. I am very fortunate to be blessed with a strong network of friends and supporters.

Joe

The preparation of BNG is a fairly demanding process for someone who is losing the ability to use his arms. It begins with the double-boiling of what looks like a pile of mulch in about six quarts of water. This is followed by a careful filtering process that requires lifting the heavy concoction and pouring it through a strainer lined with cheesecloth. The completed brew then needs to be evenly distributed into bottles in the proper amounts for daily consumption.

It didn't take long before increasing weakness of my arms made the preparation a very exhausting activity. That's when my friends, Sheryl and Richard Rosenberg, started showing up to help. Since a batch of BNG produces only about a two-week supply of the brew, we would make two or more batches at a time. Sheryl and Richard showed up loyally month after month, contributing an entire afternoon to ensure that I had a steady supply of BNG. While we couldn't do much about the pungent aroma that each brewing left lingering throughout the house (much to Diane's dismay), Sheryl and Richard made it far easier for me to stay on track with this treatment.

HEALTH UPDATE: 4/30/04

Well, the odyssey continues. My hands and arms continue to weaken, and my right leg as well. Even typing is becoming more challenging at times, with both hands tending to claw when they have had enough. Enough can be as little as a couple of short e-mails. In fact, writing this one required about four time-outs for my hands to recover. My right leg has gotten so weak that I sometimes can't move it without support from my hands. Yet, I still have enough movement in the ankle to depress the accelerator on my car, and my left foot is still at almost normal strength. So, that one takes on brake duty. Right about now, I have to imagine that some of you would like to know my driving itinerary, so you can plan to be somewhere else when I'm on the road in your area. Not to worry: The minute I feel the slightest loss of control of the vehicle, I promise to hang up my license.

OK, so now for the bad news. ONLY KIDDING—BREATHE, BREATHE!

At the moment, despite the increased weakness, I am still managing to navigate on foot using my canes and walker, and into the car. When I have to go any distance, I find someone to help propel the wheelchair. It does a lot for my mental health that I still have my independence.

One of the biggest daily challenges is getting fed, particularly with my dietary restrictions. Eating the right things to properly fuel my body and keep my weight up is critically important. I can't rely on prepared foods, and preparing meals can be extremely draining. Cutting vegetables and stirring the contents of pots can be exhausting. The cavalry is on the way to help with this issue, however.

A group of friends from my synagogue is going to take turns preparing dinners a couple of times a week until school is out and Diane is home for the summer. The long hours required by Diane's job have been an added obstacle to the support she can give me, which is enormous when she is around. The kids have been pitching in more and more, as well. So, the support network is doing its job.

Of late, I have also been doing better at getting to bed earlier, so I can still get a lot of sleep and be up earlier in the day. It takes so much

effort, time and energy just to get started in the
morning that I find myself with much shorter days.
Combine that with the extra time and effort needed
to do just about everything, and it's hard to feel
like I get much accomplished during any given day.
I am still working on shifting my expectations to
meet the current reality. It will come in time.

On the treatment front, I continue to explore
additional modes of intervention. Currently under
investigation are cold laser therapy and an
additional form of frequency treatment. I'll let
you know when something significant develops. I
continue to benefit from contact and guidance from
Dr. Kessler in Germany. Diane and I will both be
traveling there to see him again at the end of
July. Donations of airline points have continued
flowing in to help defray the costs of these
visits. I am truly blessed with some very generous
friends.

The primary treatment I am currently using
continues to be the Chinese herbal concoction
known as BNG, referred to in my last update. I
have stopped pretty much everything else for now,
except for watching the food intolerances and
avoiding toxins. By the way, recent testing
indicates that my mercury levels have come down
over 50%—so there really appears to be some
effectiveness to the frequency treatment. For now,
I am relying on the BNG for both continued
detoxification and addressing the ALS directly. I
have been on it for eight weeks, as of this
writing. So far, I am having what the study
coordinator describes as the "classic reaction,"
which unfortunately can involve significant

weakening during the first couple of months of use. During the first ninety days, what they hope to achieve is stabilization of the illness. That could begin to occur any day now. The continued weakening described earlier could very well be the early effects of the BNG draining energy from my body for use in repairing neurons, rather than progression of the ALS.

On the plus side of the ledger, since beginning the use of BNG there has been almost no cramping. Prior to starting on this protocol, I would get painful stomach spasms while trying to tie my shoes or pull on a sock. Also, my biceps would frequently cramp after a workout at the gym. These things have become rare occurrences over the last two months—almost non-existent. In addition, there are some ALS symptomatic responses that did not show up in my last examination with the motor-neuron specialist. One of them, the Bibinski reflex, was the symptom that caused my first motor-neuron specialist to confirm the ALS diagnosis last May. On April 22, it came up as negative, meaning I no longer have that response. If it continues to be absent, that is a small sign of positive change in my condition. So, stay tuned!

The contractor should be breaking ground for our new bedroom within the next four to six weeks and hopes to be done sometime in August. Diane and I are going through the joyful task of selecting fixtures for the wheelchair-accessible bathroom. I will really be glad when this is over. I also want to thank those of you who have generously contributed to the Congregational Assistance Fund at my synagogue. It has helped significantly in dealing with the growing costs of making our home a more handicapped-friendly environment.

So, the journey continues and the will stays strong. Friends, family, and people that I don't even know well continue to reach out with support in so many ways that I am almost convinced they have me confused with somebody else. My optimism remains high that I may soon be sending you updates that contain more information about improving strength and physical capabilities, than about the challenges of getting through the day. When that update comes, please remember that you have played a huge role in bringing it about just by staying interested in how I am doing. Thanks so much for caring.

Joe

These health updates describe some elements of the progression over time, and were usually focused on intention and hope. On a daily basis, however, the experience could take on a starker character.

A year after my confirmed diagnosis, my mornings were taking on a very different quality than what I had enjoyed pre-ALS. I have always loved being up early. It makes the day longer and gives me more time to accomplish things. I also find it to be the most peaceful, and often the most beautiful part of the day. There is little in life that surpasses the beauty and inspiration of the sunrise on a clear morning, framed by the majestic green stillness of mature trees, the sunlight glistening off their dew-drenched leaves, and the birds offering up their subtle symphony to welcome the dawn.

The fatigue factor from ALS, however, changed my focus. Now the simple activities of getting up, toileted, and dressed—physical movements previously taken for granted and performed unconsciously—were becoming laborious and requiring more preparation and concentration. I'd begin with a number of stretching and lifting exercises to help get the blood flowing and loosen the muscles up, preparing my body to move a little more easily. While doing the exercises, I'd take inventory, checking carefully, trying to feel something moving with less or more difficulty than it had the day before, and hoping—against the odds—to find a hint of renewed strength. Could I lift the big toe further? Could I raise my foot? Was I still able to touch the thumb and pinky on my left hand? No change? That's good. Positive change? That's the dream I long to have come true.

Hunched over and grasping onto furniture and walls for stability, I'd make my way to the bathroom. The handheld plastic shower head, installed months ago to make the job easier, now felt like it was made of lead as I guided the water over my body while seated on a shower stool. Completing the final rinse and drained from the effort, I'd sit for a few minutes trying to find more energy to reach for the towel and extract myself from the shower stall. It confounds me still how something so simple could be so exhausting. My thoughts vacillated between entertaining how easy it would be to give in, and spurring myself on to not give up. I had to keep moving. If I stopped, it would be over.

Then came the pills and the injections, followed by breakfast. Sounds like simple stuff. The problem is that, while I was performing these tasks of daily living, the weakness in my hip-flexor muscles created the feeling that I was working with a 25-pound weight hanging from my neck. Standing upright while slicing an apple required the level of energy that it would take to lift and hold an eight-year-old child over my head. The longer it took to complete the task, the more I'd find myself leaning forward, supporting myself on the kitchen counter and hunching over with the strain. Given the erosion of my fine motor skills, grasping the pieces of fruit I was cutting was like trying to pick up slippery pieces of mercury.

Why not just do the task sitting down? Sometimes, I did. If I did it all the time, however, I would risk promoting more atrophy. It was a battle worth fighting.

After breakfast and reading the paper, I resumed my therapy and then, finally, I'd be ready to get onto the computer and research treatments, work on the finances, or run some errands. On a good day, I would actually get out of the house before noon, with all of the getting-my-day-started activities actually done.

It is hard to write about this stuff without sounding a little beaten by it. And, since I have written this account over time, my state of mobility continues to evolve—some, but not all for the better. Yet, I will find strength in what I've described here, because, even though all of these activities were difficult, they were doable without assistance. Having completed the morning routine, I was still able to get into my car and do errands, drive myself to doctor's appointments, or whatever. With the help of canes and walkers and other assistive devices, my independence was still intact.

The physical challenges I just described show my status one year after my confirmed diagnosis, and four years after the onset of my symptoms. With a little luck and some help from the Almighty, my hope was to still have that independence four years hence. I prayed that, if it was lost, I would at least have the ability to maintain a constructive focus and continue the search for a way to beat this thing. My prayers were not ignored, but by the summer of 2004, my upper body strength had diminished to the point that using a walker or cane, or even getting around in a manual wheelchair, was becoming quite difficult. I took advantage of an opportunity to purchase a van that was already outfitted with a motorized scooter and lift.

HEALTH UPDATE: 8/5/04

Sorry it has taken me so long to get this update out. I was hoping to be able to report that I was scheduled for dancing lessons and a backpacking trip by now, but alas the reversal of symptoms continues to elude me. My hands, arms and legs are weaker still. Walking has become incredibly difficult, and the growing deformity and weakness in my right hand make things like writing, typing, bathing, and eating increasingly challenging.

OK, so much for the uplifting opening. There is positive news to report, however. Since acquiring the van and scooter, my mobility has been greatly increased. It allows me to take walks with Diane and to do my own errands and shopping with far greater ease. While trips to the gym have grown far less frequent, I have been able to significantly increase the number of repetitions that I can do on my bicep curls. Dropping all the way back to just ten pounds in each hand for this exercise has resulted in far more endurance on the reps during my last two or three workouts. This experience has not been consistent with other muscle groups during my workouts, though. The shoulders and forearms continue to slowly weaken, and I have already commented on my hands and legs. Yet, chewing, swallowing, and breathing remain free of difficulty, and I am still driving and getting around independently. I have also managed to put back on about five pounds.

Having Diane home for the summer has been wonderful. She has been keeping me well fed and doing a lot of schlepping and fetching to help me conserve energy. Just getting to see her more and be with her more has also made life a lot more enjoyable. I'm not looking forward to her going back to work next month.

Construction on the new addition is finally under way. The frame, walls, and roof are done. Soon, work will begin on the interior. We are hoping for completion by the end of September. Friends have pitched in to defray some of the costs by taking down part of the deck, and by offering to help out with painting when the structure is completed. Many of you have been very generous in your efforts to help with the financial burdens. I feel truly blessed. Thank you so much.

> Of all the people we know, you possess the most perseverance. When I did your travel arrangements, you would always come up with all the possibilities and never left a stone unturned.
>
> **TOBIE AND STAN**
> LONGTIME FRIENDS

Now for the breaking news— Diane and I returned from Germany this past weekend, where we both went through another round of treatment with Dr. Kessler. The news is not earth shattering in terms of any immediate changes in my physical capabilities, but we discovered a number of things that hold encouragement and promise. First, my leaky gut (a condition that interferes with proper absorption of nutrients in the colon) is now healed, and the intolerances for gluten and lactose are gone. While I still need to be conservative about consuming these substances, it indicates some concrete progress in strengthening my system and makes getting fed a whole lot easier. The cruel irony is that Diane now has to avoid milk products, fructose and fruit. So, now it's my turn to read labels for her.

The most exciting development was that Kessler provided both of us with a device called a Quint box. This is a companion piece to the Quint system that he uses for diagnosis and treatment. The box, a small device that I wear on a belt, is programmed with a variety of frequencies specifically targeted to treat the issues that were discovered during my visit to the clinic. This, in essence, enables me to receive treatment 24/7. In just the first few days of use, it has already restored warmth and improved circulation in my lower right leg and cut down the number of interruptions to my sleep during the night. A major finding in Kessler's assessment this time was that the leading disturbance in my body appears to be coming from parasites. The number-one intruder is Ricketsia, an organism known to be transmitted through tick bites. Frequencies in the Quint box will rid me of these freeloaders. Stay tuned. This could be big.

In addition to the Kessler treatment, BNG remains part of my protocol. This is my sixth month of involvement with the Chinese herbal brew, a time by which many users start to experience significant results. Keep those prayers coming! I have also begun working with a doctor of Chinese medicine in Princeton, Dr. Xie, who diagnosed me as having Wai Syndrome. This is a blockage of Chi energy channels that she has experience in correcting with acupuncture and herbs. By sometime in October, she believes she will be able to give me a better assessment of how much lost functioning she can restore. The fact that she thinks she can restore any of it is pretty amazing.

We are considering two additional treatments for some time down the road. One is through a guy in southern New York State, who has developed a machine that generates massive amounts of negative ions. He has had some amazing success in promoting healing in people with autoimmune issues and bacterial and viral diseases. Two of the leading theories on what causes ALS are autoimmune dysfunction and a viral attack on the neurons. So, this treatment could possibly have some major impact. Unfortunately, there is no experience in using it with ALS to date.

The other possibility is a procedure developed at Rutgers University and expanded upon by a Dr. Huang when he returned to China. Over the past few years, Dr. Huang has performed this procedure on over 400 cases of spinal cord injury in which he injects olfactory glial cells (whatever the heck that means) obtained from aborted fetuses into the spinal cord of the injured patients. These cells have an extraordinary ability to attach to and replace damaged neurons and to resist rejection from the patient. He has had impressive results in restoring lost function with these patients. About a year ago, he began doing a variation of the procedure for patients with ALS. This procedure includes injections in the frontal lobes of the brain! Again, his results restoring lost function for patients with ALS are proving to be pretty amazing. The procedure costs between $22,000 and $25,000 and requires a month-long stay in Beijing, along with a caregiver companion. Given the newness of the procedure, the unknown side effects and durability of the results, the scariness of having someone poking needles into my gray matter (although, some of you might think that would be helpful), and the cost in both time and money, I'm not quite ready to book a flight to Beijing. But the early results are compelling, and I will be following developments with the procedure. Dr. Huang is also very interested in the combined

effects of his procedure and BNG. So, those of us
using the herbal brew can be fast-tracked for the
procedure if we choose to pursue it. Steve Byer,
the BNG study coordinator, has been keeping the
BNG users up to date on developments. His son Ben,
who has ALS, is recovering from this procedure as
I write.

Well, I wish I had something more interesting to
report. (Hey, wake up! I'm almost done here!) But
this will have to tide you over for now.

                                        Joe

By the summer of 2004, I had acquired a power wheelchair
through the loaner program of the Philadelphia chapter of the ALS
Association. Having access to this loaner program is an incredible gift,
as these power chairs cost upwards of $20,000. The chair made
navigation around the house much easier. Outside, I was still using my
walker and scooter to get around.

My manual dexterity, which had always been one of my
strengths, had become increasingly impaired, as the capacity for
movement in my hands and arms continued to erode. Things like
opening and filing the mail had become nearly impossible. To get my
paperwork done, I had been relying on private health aides and friends
who volunteered their time to help me keep down the costs.

By the fall of 2004, my strength and fine-motor skills had
diminished to the point that I was having significant difficulty
completing some of the basic tasks of daily living. Inserting key rings
and pull-strings on zippers to poke my weakened fingers through was
barely enough to enable me to fasten my pants independently. My
Velcro-fastened sneakers, which had eliminated the impossible task of
tying a shoelace, now also required more strength than remained in my
fingers and hands. Hygiene tasks, like showering, had become either
dangerous or too difficult to manage completely on my own. The

regular expense of home health aides for a few hours each morning could no longer be avoided.

In October 2004, Diane, Dan, Julie, and I traveled to Miami for the wedding of my nephew, Michael. The weekend turned out to be an emotional roller coaster. The plan was for Michael and Dawn to be married in a hotel, followed by an afternoon meal. After that, about three-dozen family members and friends were to accompany them on an extended weekend cruise to Nassau in the Bahamas. Well, the plan went off pretty much as anticipated except for one little ALS related interruption....

Arrangements had been made for us to travel from my mother-in-law Bess's house to the airport, along with Bess, her youngest daughter, Eileen, and Eileen's four children. Shortly after we arrived at Bess's house, I began to feel faint. When the situation did not improve after about twenty minutes, we urged everyone else to head off to the airport, while Diane followed the ambulance that was transporting me to the local hospital. After about two hours of drawing blood and running a lot of expensive tests, the emergency room doctor determined I had simply become dehydrated. Unfortunately, by the time that conclusion had been reached, it was too late to catch a flight to Miami.

When Dan called later to check in on how I was doing, we told him to relax—that I appeared to be okay. We also told him to let everybody know that things were under control, and that Mom and I would be catching a flight in the morning. While we did catch a morning flight, we were unable to get there until after the ceremony. Although very disappointed, we caught up with the group just in time to board the cruise ship and join them for the weekend festivities.

A rented scooter helped me get around on the ship, and, in the few days that followed, my children, nieces, and nephews took turns pushing me around the beaches on manual wheelchairs. The most memorable activity of the weekend was when we rented a couple of boats to take about twenty of us to a secluded area for snorkeling. After gearing me up with a mask, snorkel, fins, and life jacket, Dan and Michael gently lowered me into the water and assisted me in grabbing onto a plastic raft that had been provided by our guides. We quickly discovered that my legs no longer had the strength to propel me in any sustained way through the water. But just as quickly as we discovered the problem, Dan and Michael provided a solution. Flanking me, they grabbed the ends of the raft, allowing the strength of their legs to provide the locomotion that my own legs could not.

The water was about fifteen feet deep, crystal clear and teeming with an amazing array of aquatic life. One of the guides dove to the bottom and used a prod to chase a huge multi-colored crustacean out into the open for us to see. As we drifted gently through the water, taking in the colorful display of sea life, I was thrilled to be participating in one of my favorite pastimes once again. Among my most powerful memories of that day was the overwhelming sense of love and support that I was feeling from the two young men beside me who were making it all possible.

> Joe once saved my life! We were abalone diving in the Pacific Ocean and I got stuck in a rip current with only one swim fin and an injured knee. Just when I thought I was about to be swept into the rock cliffs, Joe and my brother-in-law appeared on an inflatable raft, surprised to see me. With their good legs, they paddled me out of the current and safely to shore—joking all the way of course.
>
> **RICHARD LUIBRAND**
> **FAMILY FRIEND**

HEALTH UPDATE: 12/17/04

Happy Holidays! There are basically two reasons for the long dry spell between updates. One is that my typing ability has pretty much degenerated to the cumbersome two-fingered hunt and peck method. Combined with a tendency for my hands to cramp up, this has turned the longer e-mails into quite a chore. The other reason is that I still haven't achieved a breakthrough, which makes it more difficult to find fresh things to write about. However, never having been accused of having too little to say, I will persevere, secure in the knowledge that you can always hit the delete button if you're not finding the update useful.

Let's start out with the status of my functioning. I can no longer safely balance my weight and take a step without a cane or a walker, and there isn't enough strength left in my hands, arms, and shoulders to stabilize myself with the canes. So, now I'm pretty much getting around with walkers and wheelchairs.

The completion of our addition in October has made life much easier. In addition to more roaming space for the electric wheelchair, it gives me easy access to my bed, clothes, and bathroom. I am still able to drive short distances, when the weather permits. Cold and precipitation make it harder to function, and increase the difficulty of gaining access to my car and scooter. I am still handling most of my own personal hygiene, with my home health aide or family members helping out when needed. Dressing myself is an onerous task, but still mostly doable, except for socks and shoes. I could do that myself if necessary, but I would probably need a nap to recover from the effort.

OK, given that this may be more information than some of you need, let's shift slightly. The best news with regard to my functioning is that there is still little evidence of decline in critical functions like chewing, swallowing, and breathing. While my lung capacity is slightly diminished, it is still almost normal and nowhere near cause for alarm.

Trips to the gym have pretty much stopped. Between the time and effort it takes to get there, weakness and cramping interfering with physical movement as simple as lifting a fork, and the time needed for naps and meditation, it just doesn't work for me anymore. My health aide helps me get through physical therapy exercises in the morning to maintain range of motion, but that and the effort required for activities of daily living are about all the exercise I can manage. My weight seems to have stabilized at around 145. So, at least I've stopped impersonating the incredible disappearing man.

With Diane back to the enormous demands of her work schedule, she isn't around much these days. She puts in a lot of effort on weekends and the occasional weeknights she gets to be home. Our kids and friends pick up a lot of the slack making sure I get fed, get to doctor appointments, and helping out with paperwork. So far, I have been able to avoid the expense of more home-health-aide hours.

On the treatment front, I am heading back to Germany next month, this time with my son, Dan. BNG, while it may have been helping to slow the progression, has neither stopped the disease nor reversed any weakness. I will be taking an extended break from it starting in January. Acupuncture treatments continue to increase my energy, but have yet to translate into increased strength. I am stepping up meditation and napping efforts in an attempt to get more from the acupuncture. These combined strategies have worked for others and still hold promise for me. I also continue to use the Quint Box and look forward to getting the programming for it updated.

I have not yet tried the mega-negative ion machine. That may still be an option down the road. Dr. Huang's glial cell procedure in China has not produced impressive enough results to convince me that it is worth the costs in time, money, and stress—not to mention the risk of having them poke those needles too far into my brain! Other potential options continue to emerge. We'll see what develops.

The most exciting thing that has developed with treatment is a heightened awareness of the incredible importance of rest, meditation, and the way I think about the disease. To facilitate my efforts to do more with naps and meditation, I have gotten some expert help. Through the coming together of a variety of inputs, it recently occurred to me that the way I have been thinking about my situation may very well hold the key to getting more from treatment. Here's how it plays out. I have pretty consistently held to the notion throughout this ordeal that recovery (at some level) is a possibility. The flaw in this way of thinking is that, if reversing this disease is a "possibility," then the opposite is also a "possibility." ALS is a neurological disorder, and the brain is the center of the nervous system. If my brain is sending out messages to the rest of the system that recovery is only an "option," not a given, then potential for recovery has been compromised. So, my strategy going forward is to be convinced that recovery is a certainty, and that it has already begun.

For those of you to whom this may sound a little too "woo-wooish," and who may be concerned that I have totally lost it, let me assure you that the logical/rational functioning of my mind is still intact. The problem is that the logical/rational traditional approach to dealing with ALS offers little hope, and that doesn't work for me. So, while I continue to explore new paths for beating this thing, I ask that you put aside your skepticism and send me lots of positive energy based on the conviction that I will recover. I feel strongly that once my brain is convinced that it can orchestrate recovery, it will happen, and the results of healing will become visible.

Well, that pretty much sums up the current situation. You know the rest—about the journey continuing, and the will staying strong, yaddah, yaddah, yaddah (did I spell that right?).... The thing that continues to be most amazing is the incredible lesson in humanity that this experience has presented. I will never be able to adequately express the enormous level of gratitude I feel toward my family and friends for all that you do to support me in this quest. I still look forward to writing to you about getting back into golf—or hiking, tennis, skiing, and maybe even dancing lessons (I threw that last one in for Diane).

Joe

The BNG adventure lasted about nine months, from March to December 2004. As it was actually part of an informal study, I was asked to submit bi-weekly reports on various aspects of my physical, emotional, and psychological status. These reports included things like changes in weight, strength, and mood. At the beginning of my adventure, I weighed about 145 pounds (a good forty pounds lighter than my normal weight of 185). During the time I was using BNG, I experienced an easing of muscular cramping and rigidity and some modest weight gain (about five pounds), but remained unsuccessful in halting the erosion of my muscle strength. Despite the cases I had heard about in which people had achieved significant symptom reversal using BNG, it was becoming quite clear that I was not destined for these kinds of results. By the final month, I was beginning to experience flu-like detox symptoms. The intensity of these symptoms, combined with the continued decline in muscle strength, led me to conclude that it was time to move on.

My rendezvous with the mega-negative ion machine never occurred. It turned out that the inventor had it set up in his basement, which was down a long, narrow flight of stairs. At that point in time, my condition was such that I couldn't figure out a way to gain access. Whether the machine could have had any positive effect will forever remain a mystery.

CHAPTER EIGHT:
Struggling to Stay Hopeful

Upon returning from my final visit to Germany in January 2005, I found myself struggling with the probability that I had grown too weak to repeat the trip. Exhaustion from the travel had wiped out any gains from the treatment. I continued at home with Kessler's protocol, as was typical, for the next five or six months, following his guidance through phone conversations and e-mails. With BNG and acupuncture already on hold, the thought of not being able to return to Germany left me very uneasy about what I might do next. It had been five years since the onset of my symptoms. At this point, there were no other options in sight.

HEALTH UPDATE: 2/21/05

It's time for another update, to reveal the results of my recent trip to Germany.

My typing ability is still at the two-fingered hunt-and-peck level, with the additional challenge of an increase in the frequency and severity of hand cramping and fatiguing. So, if you e-mail me—and please don't hesitate to do so—be patient in waiting for a response, since keeping up with e-mail can be quite cumbersome at times.

As for the rest of my functioning, let's start with the good news. I am still able to feed myself most of the time, operate a keyboard, shave, brush my own teeth, turn pages well enough to read a newspaper or book, get doors opened and closed, operate light switches, and transfer myself to and from chairs and vehicles. There are probably a few more things I have left out, but just how much of a list like this can you tolerate!?

On the downside, all of the things in the previous list take enormous effort and sap my energy to the point that it is necessary to take frequent rest breaks. Showering and dressing independently are no longer possible. Driving is no longer safe, and I have not been able to scale the six steps from the den to the kitchen since returning from Germany in late January. The trip, while worth the effort, took a lot out of me, leaving me noticeably weaker than when I left—the inability to climb the steps being one clear example. We are in the process of acquiring a stair glide to help me regain access to the kitchen, deck, and dining room. I am spending most of my time in wheelchairs, walking only occasionally with walkers to transfer between chairs and vehicles. Visiting other homes now requires advance planning for access to the house and to a bathroom. I am working on acquiring some portable ramps to make access in other homes more manageable.

> "Daddy Joe is a fighter, someone dedicated not only to living, but to having a life; someone who loves his family and has dedicated that life to them; patient; someone who doesn't lose his head when everything around him falls apart; strong, sensitive...
>
> **LAUREN LARSON**
> **CLOSE FRIEND OF JULIE**

Happily, there is still little evidence of decline in critical functions like chewing, swallowing, and breathing. While my lung capacity feels slightly more diminished, I won't know for sure

until my next motor-neuron check-up on March 3,
and it remains at a level that is nowhere near
cause for alarm. The one thing that does generate
a little concern is a tickling sensation in my
throat that comes and goes, interrupting my
speaking and breathing with the irritation it
causes. Hopefully, this is nothing more than the
recurrence of a dry throat condition that I
developed years ago as a professional hazard from
frequent speaking assignments.

With the cold weather being hard to tolerate, I
have been spending a lot of time indoors this
winter. Friends and an additional health aide, who
is able to provide flexible hours, have been
helping me make some progress on thinning out
files and keeping up with mail, while also
assisting with meals and meds when Diane and the
kids are not around. I have even managed to
continue doing a limited amount of pro-bono
coaching, mainly to keep my skills sharp, and to
make sure that I am still being useful.

I continue to feel incredibly blessed with the
overwhelming support from friends and family, who
do everything from fix-it jobs around the house to
helping with meals, opening mail, and assisting
with personal stuff that you really don't want to
read about. It's impossible to find words to
adequately express my gratitude and appreciation.

I want to acknowledge my son (Dan), my wife
(Diane), and my daughter (Julie) for the enormous
effort they put in contributing to my care in the
midst of very busy schedules. Diane leaves for
work at 6:00 a.m. and is frequently not home until
10:00 p.m. She continues to work the magic that

has earned her a reputation as one of the best choral directors in the state. Dan is busily and successfully building his career as a musician, racing each week from playing piano at Nordstrom's to teaching French horn to nearly a dozen students, while playing horn in several local orchestras and gigging frequently on both horn and piano. He manages this hectic schedule in addition to ongoing audition preparation for spots in summer festivals and horn openings in major orchestras. Julie, now represented by two New York modeling agencies, is making frequent treks into the city for auditions. Meanwhile, she is babysitting her brains out to keep money coming in until the modeling gigs blossom into a full career. In the midst of these demanding schedules, they never fail to provide their time when I need it, and they do it with a degree of love and care that fills me with pride and awe. Dan's care-giving in Germany is a shining example.

Dan accompanied me on the January trip to the Kessler Clinic. He wheeled, fed, shaved, and bathed me, and even carried me when needed. Moreover, he did it without complaint, and with a love and tenderness that had me frequently choking back tears. My caring and supportive family is a huge source of strength and inspiration. I am blessed, and I am grateful beyond words.

OK, quick Kleenex break.... Now, back to current treatment.

BNG is no longer in the current mix. I tried for nine months but just couldn't warm up to the taste. And it also wasn't producing the hoped-for results. In addition, we discovered some evidence while in Germany that it may have been interfering with Kessler's treatment. So, while another try is a possibility, it is currently out of the picture.

Acupuncture treatments are also currently on hold after a five-month trial. While each treatment seemed to produce a short-lived boost of energy, the increases were neither sustained nor translated into restored strength. After discussions with Drs. Xie and Kessler, the three of us agreed that it made sense to suspend acupuncture as well, and to focus completely on Kessler's protocol for the next few months.

I have been successful at building afternoon naps and meditation into my routine, and this will continue. It never ceases to amaze me how much of a difference these things make in sustaining energy and strength, and how much I suffer for it when the practice is omitted! I've decided to keep doing these things even after recovery. We could learn a lot from other cultures, where they practice things like siestas—even when they are healthy.

The assessment during my week with Kessler revealed, as usual, that some things have improved, while new issues have been clarified. A disappointing finding was that none of the issues identified during my last visit, in July, have been completely resolved. Kessler commented that, since he began using the Quint Box with his patients, this is the first time he has seen that happen. This finding was the key reason for his suspicions that the BNG might have been interfering. On the plus side, he believes that the current issues we are treating may represent the last layer of factors contributing to the paralysis and blocking my body from healing itself. So, the hope is that I can remain stable enough and strong enough to return to Germany this summer, and that there will be little left to work on. If this plays out and my body starts to heal, then I could begin to regain strength sometime later this year.

Before you jump too high for joy over this prospect, please keep in mind that there has been significant, albeit slow loss of strength over the past six months. I have been working diligently with doctor Kessler through phone and e-mail discussions, making ongoing adjustments to both the new Quint Box programs and the dosage of the suitcase full of homeopathic remedies with which I returned. My body was being overwhelmed, at first, by the sheer volume of remedies. Things have now begun to settle down. Hopefully, results are not too far away. If the Kessler protocol does not work, there are still a variety of interventions to explore. It will simply mean choosing the next plan of attack.

I truly appreciate the encouragement I got from many of you over the brain-retraining effort I wrote about in the last update. It is certainly no small task to convince yourself that you are in recovery from a degenerative disease while you are clearly observing your physical capabilities erode. The feedback from your calls and e-mails that I was not being too "woo-woo" was re-assuring, and strengthened my resolve to stay the course.

Yesterday, I had the unfortunate need to attend a memorial service. It was for a man named Harvey Tesser. Harvey was the man most responsible for founding and nurturing into existence the synagogue in which I have proudly held membership for the past nineteen years. He was a forceful and determined man, who occasionally rubbed people the wrong way (as strong personalities often do). He was also both a visionary and a doer, who had the persistence to drive his visions to reality. You just had to respect the man, and I did—deeply. We had worked closely together as board members years ago, and I thought that I knew him reasonably well. As I listened to his children, grandchildren, wife, business associates, and friends lovingly eulogize him in front of the standing room-only crowd, though, it occurred to me that there was much more to this man than I had been privileged to know. I felt awed and a little cheated that there were so many wonderful things about Harvey to which I had not been exposed. I couldn't help but wonder and hope that he knew in life how these people felt about him.

As Diane and I drove home, it was impossible not to reflect on how this scene might play out for me when the time comes. Diane was quick to point out that regardless of what will happen when I'm gone, the people who care about me display it continuously, through an endless stream of support in the form of phone calls, e-mails, meals, home maintenance help, office help, driving me to doctor appointments, running errands, monetary contributions, and more. Now, this doesn't mean that I don't still expect you to show up in droves and say wonderful things about me (even if you have to make stuff up!) when that day comes. But I want to thank you for helping to keep my quality of life feeling rich and rewarding.

Joe

In the meantime, while Dr. Xie had been successful in reversing symptoms with a limited number of ALS-diagnosed patients, I did not appear destined to become her latest success story. I left each visit feeling more energized and slightly stronger, but the progress of each visit evaporated by the next one—we could not achieve a cumulative effect. After five months of trying, she concluded that some sort of energy blockage was preventing our progress, and that something else was needed. It was disappointing that we could not replicate some of her past success, but our relationship was far from over.

Diane's comments about how people have rallied to my aid really struck home. It occurred to me that this support was evident even in response to the health updates. In response to each update, I have typically received two or three dozen e-mails, including messages of support, admiration, and encouragement. Additionally, these e-mails have often contained information useful in pursuing my health goals. It is simply not possible to put into words what these responses have meant. The feedback has provided valuable perspective on how I am dealing with the situation. It has served as an immeasurable source of strength, which has helped me remain positive and focused on the quest for recovery.

The stair glide mentioned previously, which was acquired through the loaner program of the New York chapter of the ALS Association, enabled me to get upstairs to the kitchen, dining room, and deck area, where we kept a manual wheelchair to help me get around on that level. My friend Gil had attached a wooden platform with wheels to the bottom of an old bar stool, which enabled me to navigate around the kitchen with access to the countertops. Pushing myself around the kitchen on this contraption with the remaining strength in my legs had preserved my ability to do much of my own food preparation. I had been using this wheeled stool for about a year, but the weakness in my hands was now making it more difficult to manage knives and cooking utensils. Food preparation was another task of daily living that was about to be turned over to a health aide, further diminishing both my independence and my bank account.

HEALTH UPDATE: 5/16/05

At the risk of starting out on a sour note, I am sorry to report that there isn't much in the way of uplifting news since the February update. My breathing capacity has eroded down to about 50 percent. About six weeks ago, I began using something called a Bi-PAP machine to assist my breathing while I sleep. A cough-assist machine is now used to remove unwanted food particles, which I no longer have the strength to cough up, from my throat and lungs. For the past month, I have been sleeping in a hospital bed, having lost the ability to sit up and lift myself out of a regular bed. We are in the process of looking for a wheelchair-accessible van, because the process of transferring between wheelchairs, car seats, and my scooter is becoming increasingly challenging, time-consuming, and risky.

Typing ability is devolving into a one-fingered hunt-and-peck, because I now need to support one hand with the other while moving a finger around the keyboard. The recent acquisition of a keyboard tray attached to an extended swivel arm has made it possible to position the keyboard over the reclined wheelchair, providing more support for my head, neck, and arms. I have also recently discovered that Windows XP has an on-screen keyboard available in its accessibility file, which makes typing a little more manageable. I can type from my lap with a mouse and mouse pad, using a narrower range of motion. This takes the strain off my arms, but is still somewhat fatiguing for my hands.

As for the rest of my functioning, again let's start with the good news. While Emily Post might not approve of my technique, I am still able to feed myself most of the time. Brushing my teeth and combing my hair are still doable but extremely difficult. Similarly, turning pages is still possible, although with considerable effort. My abilities to open and close doors, operate light switches, and transfer myself to and from chairs and vehicles remain about the same. The stair glide has been installed, restoring my access to living areas. We have also acquired portable ramps, making visits to friends more manageable, but we are finding that it is usually easier having a few people get together and carry me inside in my wheelchair. All of these activities take enormous effort and sap my energy, as you know. Even shaving requires so much effort that I now let my health aide do most of the work.

Hey, I promised to keep you up to date, but I can't always promise good news. It kind of puts the daily annoyances most of us complain about into perspective, though, doesn't it?

Treatment remains focused on Kessler's work in Germany, with the hope that the final obstacles to recovery are being addressed, and that the beginning of a turnaround is not far away. As Tug McGraw, of the 1969 Amazin' Mets, was fond of saying, "You gotta believe!" We are trying to figure out how to get back to Germany this summer without breaking the bank, while avoiding the physical stress that sapped so much of my strength during the January trip. I am searching for a homeopathic sleeping pill and an affordable way of flying business class so I can sleep on the plane. The potential loss of function from the physical strain of flying coach again is something I don't even want to think about. Unfortunately, the costs of business class are outrageous, and the financial strain is compounded by the impending purchase of my wheelchair-accessible van. So, I may have to pass up further treatment from Kessler and move on to something else. It would be disappointing to have to move on without knowing if the work there was complete, but what can ya do?

Joe

To be honest, the net gains from Kessler's treatment were hard to assess. I strongly believe that there was great benefit, both physical and psychological, despite the fact that my body continued to deteriorate during the course of that treatment. The concrete gains—like reduction in pesticides, heavy metals, and other toxins at the cellular level and the healing of a leaky gut that improved my digestion—were not clearly visible to the human eye, but only detectable through testing with instrumentation. With Kessler's treatment, acupuncture and BNG all having failed to produce the desired results, it was beginning to feel like the walls were closing in. My search for a treatment that could yield tangible, observable reversal of physical symptoms would have to continue along another road. The trouble was, I had no idea what that road would be or how to find it.

CHAPTER NINE

Closed Chapters, New Opportunities

The Dance of Detox

By the summer of 2005, six months after that last trip to Germany, I was beginning to feel a little desperate. I was unable to drive, dependent on a walker and motorized scooter for my mobility, unable to navigate stairs, and still slowly deteriorating. The most alarming change, from a medical perspective, was that my breathing capacity had dropped below the 40 percent level, making me eligible for hospice. At the urging of my neurologist, I enrolled, gaining access to the vast resources this organization provides. Most important among these was the additional home health care that, as a hospice patient, my insurance would cover.

Despite the advantages of engaging with hospice, admission into the program presented a huge psychological hurdle. The inescapable reality is that a person cannot be accepted into hospice unless a case can be made by the physician that the patient's life expectancy is likely to be six months or less. Here I was, trying to convince my brain that I was in fact in recovery, and yet I had signed up for a program that labeled me as someone for whom the clock was ticking— rapidly. I was eventually able to get past this dreadful implication, but it was no small thing to overcome. Not

> I have often been accused of being somewhat compulsive with a strong Meyers Briggs "J"...but my need for closure pales in comparison to Joe.
>
> The good news about that was always knowing he could be counted on to be "buttoned up" as a consultant. I never thought twice about Joe's ability to nail down any assignment.
>
> It's that same relentless drive, I believe, which supports him in not allowing ALS to defeat him. He is a hero to me.
>
> **HOWARD GUTTMAN**
> COLLEAGUE AND FRIEND

having a solid treatment plan in place at the time didn't make it any easier.

Around the same time that I was entering hospice, a friend of mine, who was also fighting some complicated medical issues with alternative approaches, referred me to Sue Ann Garwood, a practitioner of electro-dermal testing. Having become familiar with this technology in Germany, I was delighted to find someone versed in this process close to home. Electro-dermal testing is a simple, non-invasive procedure that uses electrodes on the hands and cuticles to determine the presence of a wide variety of toxins in the body. Four hours of testing revealed that, while some of my toxin levels had been reduced, many remained to be addressed. Sue Ann's major contribution was to refer me to another practitioner who she felt could be more helpful. Thus began my involvement with Quantum Reflex Analysis (QRA).

It was time to update my fan club on these changes in my treatment plan. I needed to find a way to let people know about hospice without scaring the hell out of them. I also wanted to acknowledge that I was reconciled to not returning to Germany, and to tell them that I had found another road to pursue. A flash of mischievous creativity led me to begin this health update as if I were narrating an episode in a soap opera. Lightening the mood with levity seemed a good way to soften the impact of the news about hospice.

HEALTH UPDATE: 7/17/05

You may recall from the last episode that Joe's breathing capacity had dipped to about the 50 percent level. Well, sadly, since last we visited him, our hero's breathing capacity has dipped further, to the 30-40 percent range. With this measurement in hand, the doctor looked him in the eye, and said, "Joe, you have a choice. We can either do a tracheostomy, or consider hospice." Joe steeled himself, looked the doctor back in the eye, and asked, "How long do you think I have, Doc?" The doctor explained that while

hospice was originally designed to help people
spend their final days in comfort and dignity,
many people survive for years on hospice care
because of the increase in the frequency and
quality of care that comes with it. Joe and his
lovely wife, Diane, pondered this information,
considered the advantages of additional home
health care and decreased insurance hassles, and
decided to sign up.

So, there you have it, people: I'm now on hospice,
still planning on being around for a while and
sticking it to this rotten disease (apparently, I
am also considering a career in writing for soap
operas). With the twenty hours per week of home
health care now provided by hospice, and the
fifteen I've been getting from ALSA, I am now
covered for seven hours each day, Monday through
Friday. This is a huge relief for us, both
physically and monetarily.

With regard to the rest of my functioning (other
than breathing), there isn't much news. I continue
to weaken, but very slowly. The search for a
wheelchair-accessible van continues. Venturing
outside the neighborhood has become more
restricted simply because it requires so much
effort, both for me and for a helper. Finding the
right van should change that.

On the treatment front, we have let go of the idea
of returning to Germany, at least for now. While I
will continue to remain in contact with Dr.
Kessler, the threat of accelerated weakening from
the stress of travel has proved too great an
obstacle. While working with Kessler from afar, I

have also recently found some resources closer to home. One of these people is a nutritionist by the name of Wendy Krasner. In addition to her work as a nutritionist, Wendy practices a methodology called Quantum Reflex Analysis (QRA). QRA involves the use of kinesiology to identify toxicities and nutrient deficiencies. This is similar to some of Kessler's work, with the added advantages of more frequent accessibility and potentially more powerful detoxing agents and nutritional supplements. I will be starting a QRA protocol this coming week. So, stay tuned for the next exciting ride!

Friends and family remain ever present and supportive. In late May, my consulting associates showed up *en masse* for a gardening party to plant shrubs and spring flowers around our addition. It was a wonderful bonding opportunity for the whole team, and a wonderful gift

---

In the spring of 2004, several students, Mrs. Martin, the orchestra teacher, and Mr. Linford, a parent of one of my students, approached me to mention that they were planning to have a benefit concert in honor of our family, to help raise funds for Joe and ALS. I am a very private person, so most of my students didn't know that Joe had been fighting ALS for over 2 years. I had thought, a couple of months prior, that the students sensed something was wrong. I received the most wonderful letter from one of them, expressing concern. "I am just another face in the choir, just another one of your many children. You have been the object of strength to us this far. Now let us return the favor. Let us help you.... Let us heal you. After all, 'Trust in the morrow, and it shall come'"—a quote from a song that we had sung that year. When I read that letter, it made me realize that my students were already sharing in our struggle, which made it easier to open up to them. And so began the start of SerenAide, the benefit concert for Joe that is still given each year to raise funds for ALS and those afflicted with the disease.

DIANE WIONS

98

for us. Also in May, Diane's students organized a benefit concert that raised a significant amount of money for the ALS Association and the Jewish Community Center of Belle Mead, the two organizations that have supported us most through this ordeal. It was a wonderful evening of music, with an outpouring of love from a community very appreciative of my wife's talents as a teacher, and her gifts to their children over the past years. The blessings never cease! Thank you all for continuing to be there for me and for my family.

Joe

Wendy Krasner had been trained in QRA by the originator of this exotic-sounding process. As I came to understand it from a client's perspective, this process uses muscle-strength testing (kinesiology) to determine organ weaknesses and then to assess the type and amount of herbal treatment with which to strengthen them. For about a year, once or twice a month, I traveled an hour and a quarter each way to be reassessed and have my protocol adjusted. The treatment included a lengthy list of herbal substances, mostly in capsule form, in addition to other regimens described in my Health Update, anti-oxidant juices, food substances, and more. I was in for quite a ride, with many ups and downs.

HEALTH UPDATE: 12/11/05

Just in case any of you were wondering, I'm still here!! My energy and movement have become so constricted and my days so filled with treatment strategies that I haven't been able to get an update out since July. So, today, with the help of my good friend, June, I'll try to bring you up to date.

Physically, the picture is mixed. I get lots of feedback on how "good" I look, despite the fact that I have become extremely challenged by activities as simple as pushing the buttons on a hand-held phone. Personally, I think people are just being kind and trying to do what they think is appropriate to help me stay positive. I look in the mirror and see a skinny guy who appears older than his years. But, I will admit that my skin has good color and a lovely, healthy glow.

As you may recall from my last note (if your long-term memory is that good), I began treatment during the summer with a nutritionist by the name of Wendy Krasner who has been using a technique called Quantum Reflex Analysis to try to eliminate the underlying causes of my illness. We have determined these to fall into three groups: parasitic infestation, viral infection, and heavy metals. After much trial and error on handling an enormously challenging treatment plan, I think we are finally starting to make some progress. We had a recent victory in eliminating liver fluke from my system, which was a major part of the parasitic infestation. We are now going after the remaining parasites and building slowly toward attacks on the viruses and metals.

The way I feel from day to day varies because of the amount of detoxing elicited by the herbs involved in the treatment. This is a good news/bad news scenario. The fact that I feel lousy at times is an indication that the intruders are being eliminated from my system. But I still feel lousy. After getting rid of the liver fluke, and before altering the protocol, I got to experience a period of much higher energy, a little increased strength, and greatly improved sleep. So, even though those results have been inconsistent since revising the protocol, I have clear evidence that this plan can make a difference. Hang in there with me for the roller-coaster ride...it could actually lead to some degree of recovery. The question is whether I can stop the deterioration of my body in time for the treatment to turn things around.

I want to extend a heartfelt thanks to all of you who helped with the purchase of my new van. Having a wheelchair-accessible vehicle has made getting around a possibility again.

Unfortunately, with the need to take multiple doses of pills each day, along with mudpacks and castor oil packs and other treatments too disgusting to mention here, I don't get a lot of time to travel. I am also incredibly indebted to the army of friends and relatives who donate their time to helping with my care on weekends. Since there is very little I can now do without assistance, it is an incredible emotional and physical drain on my wife and children to handle my care when the health aides are not around. I continue to marvel at the miracles of human kindness from which I benefit every day. Thanks again for caring, sending lots of positive energy, and being an integral part of my recovery plan. Let me also take this opportunity to wish you all a very happy and healthy holiday season and New Year.

                                        Joe

Although the acquisition of the van made getting around much more manageable, the demands of my treatment resulted in infrequent use during the first year we owned it. We spent as much time getting it repaired as we did using it for transportation. It was becoming more of a drain on our bank account than an asset for my mobility.

My experiences with QRA had become quite a roller coaster ride. The demands of the process were taking quite a toll on me, both physically and emotionally. Between the various body treatments, the pill consumption and frequent trips to the bathroom caused by the volume of water required to wash down the pills, it was difficult to find time to do anything else. The feeling of being housebound was weighing heavily on my outlook and spirits. Yet the occasional success, like the effects of eliminating the liver fluke, and the absence of any better treatment options at the time, kept me hooked into the process.

> This was a scary time for the kids and me. While Joe aimed to stay positive as he gave Wendy's treatment a fair chance, his weight and energy levels plummeted. It was very difficult for us to watch, and for Joe to experience. Wendy's protocol involved Joe taking upwards of 200 herbal pills and capsules a day. This occupied the majority of his time, and left little room for food, or any real enjoyment in life. We were experiencing a common and difficult dilemma, one we had to face multiple times throughout his illness. At what point does one give up on a treatment option? At what point are "detoxing symptoms" no longer practical?
>
> **DIANE WIONS**

HEALTH UPDATE: 4/29/06

June is back for a visit today, so I thought I'd take advantage of her typing skills and her willingness to help get out another update. I'm not getting as many compliments about how good I look. I'm not sure exactly what that means. Maybe people are just getting tired of telling me, or maybe I'm really starting to look like crap. I'm opting for the first one because when I look in the mirror, I still see the same skinny guy with the wonderful glow.

It's hard to say how much has actually changed since December. I guess that's a good thing. My breathing capacity remains in the low 20 percent range. While that's not good, it's not much of a change since December. My movement continues to become more restricted and more challenging in most ways. Yet, there have been some small indications of returned strength, like the ability to wave my left hand when seated in a reclining position. It ain't much, but I'll take whatever I can get. The last couple of months have had some scary moments, including an evening when I had so much trouble breathing that I feared I might not see daylight.

Since the victory over the liver fluke back in November, the herbal treatment plan has become increasingly challenging. The time and energy it takes has been creating a good deal of stress and limiting my food intake dramatically. As a result, I have cut back on it, increased my use of the Bi-PAP (breathing machine) with daytime naps, and increased the use of some medication that helps to reduce the twitching from my Tourette's Syndrome (another enormous energy drainer). I have also, according to my respiratory therapist, quite possibly become the first person in history to learn how to eat while having a breathing machine pumping air into his nose. But, then again, you already knew how talented I was! The result of all this is that I am experiencing fewer difficult detox reactions (maybe a good thing, maybe not), eating better, feeling less stressed about trying to pump pills down my throat, managing my energy more effectively and, occasionally, finding time to get out of the house.

My nutritionist continues to find signs of progress in the effort to detoxify my body, but not a lot of it has translated into positives about how I feel or function. There has been some decrease in pain, but that's about the only tangible evidence of progress. I still believe that the approach can be helpful, but we are working to find a less stressful way to apply it, lest the cure kill me before it heals me.

Another big change is that we now have a live-in aide. The difficulty of having three different health aides coming and going during the course of the day became far too challenging. Each time there was a change in personnel, the effort of retraining was exhausting me further. Having a live-in who gets a break in the afternoon from my hospice aide makes things a little more manageable, but I'm still dealing with training new people, which further increases the difficulty of staying on the treatment plan.

My main focus these days is working on my belief system, which I am still convinced is one of the most important keys to the possibility of recovery. I work every day at programming my brain to focus on healing the nerves and muscles. If neurological dysfunction is what causes ALS, then there's a chance that I can program better function into my nerves and give the herbs a little extra boost in their effort to get my body functioning the way it's supposed to again.

Knowing that you guys are out there caring and praying for me also continues to be a big part of what keeps me going. Next Friday, May 5, we get to experience another one of those supportive miracles that people who care about us keep creating. Diane's students at J.P. Stevens High School in Edison, NJ are running their second annual SerenAide concert to honor us and to raise money for the Philadelphia chapter of ALSA and the Jewish Community Center of Belle Mead. The first SerenAide was a highly emotional outpouring of love and music, and a total surprise. Knowing that this second one is coming, Diane is able to bring home stories of how the kids are scurrying around trying to be secretive about their preparations. The level of dedication they are displaying is both moving and inspiring. If you're in the neighborhood, please join us. It's sure to be an entertaining and heartwarming evening.

Joe

The upside of the detoxing generated by the QRA process is that my body shed large quantities of toxins and organisms that were compromising my immune system and preventing it from employing its natural abilities to heal itself. The downside was watching my weight drop to a mere 115 pounds as I ingested more than 200 capsules per day instead of food, plus my breathing capacity had dwindled to the 20 percent range. In addition, the detox symptoms could be quite hard on a body already weakened by serious illness. They had taken the form of fevers in my legs and feet, flu-like symptoms, and severe vertigo, to name a few. In the end, Wendy's treatment resulted in some modest, if sporadic, gains involving basic bodily functions, reduction of pain, improved appetite (at times) and improvement in hand strength. What it did not deliver was the sustained, consistent improvement in muscle strength that I was still determined to achieve—plus it was costing a great deal of money.

> When Joe started using the BiPAP, I became increasingly concerned with his breathing at night, and his condition in general. When a person becomes that dependent on people and machines for the most basic needs, that person can require a level of care similar to a new born baby. At night, I became a very light sleeper. During holidays and gatherings, the kids and I would multitask our social involvement with an awareness of whether Joe's chest was expanding with the BiPAP. We would eat our meals, knowing that at any moment, we might have to drop our utensils to grab the cough assist machine, should he choke or have difficulty swallowing.
>
> **DIANE WIONS**

It was now almost three years since my confirmed diagnosis. At this point, I was dependent on others for getting food into my mouth and needed to be lifted in and out of bed. The BiPAP (bilateral positive air pressure) machine, referred to in my health update, was now required to force additional air into my lungs both during sleep and throughout most of the day. I lacked the arm and hand strength to scratch an itch, rub my nose, hold a book, turn a page, hold a pen, or type on a keyboard. Typing on the computer was accomplished by dictating to others, or with the use of an on-screen keyboard and a mouse to peck out the letters one laborious click at a time. A single e-mail had become an exhausting activity, and I longed for those days when, hunched over the kitchen counter, I could still prepare my own meals.

My body was in such a weakened state that I could no longer operate a phone. This made the practice of Diane departing for work in the morning and leaving me in bed with a phone, a water bottle, and a urinal until my health aide arrived no longer tenable. By April '06, as you read in the previous health update, we were forced to hire a live-in aide to ensure around-the-clock coverage.

Had I found Wendy a year earlier, I might have benefited more from her approach. I had opportunities to talk with other clients who could verify the positive impact she was having with them. But, with the cost of her treatment and the added expense of additional home health care, the limited results could not justify continuing Wendy's protocol. I was yearning for a change in approach, and Wendy knew it.

What I most valued about Wendy was her unbounded dedication to finding ways to help her clients. While QRA was the core of her practice, she would refer clients to any treatment or process she thought could be helpful. Ultimately, it was this feature of how she operated that led me to move away from her practice.

She recommended the "lemonade diet" as a way to accelerate the cleansing of my body. The idea was to get to a point where response to the herbs would be better, and fewer of them would be required. In my weakened state, I was reluctant to give up food and live on this special lemonade concoction without the support of someone who knew what they were doing with it. That's when Wendy introduced me to Tom Woloshyn and Tamara Olson.

In the late summer of 2006, Tom and Tamara traveled 3,000 miles across the continent to move into my house for two weeks and introduce me to what seemed like the most exotic approach I had yet experienced. The lemonade diet was the core of their program. Also known as the "Master Cleanser," this regimen was originally developed by health coach and author, Stanley Burroughs, several decades ago. Like most alternative practices, it has its fair share of advocates and detractors, but the success stories I learned about provided enough motivation to commit to a first trial of fifty consecutive days of fasting on lemons, water, and a few other ingredients.

To accelerate the cleansing even further, I was introduced to a Colema Board. This involved a process similar to colonics, but using a special brew of herbs in the water and a process that is controlled by the user, not a practitioner. In support of my efforts, Diane, Dan and Julie all decided to join me in this treatment.

For ten consecutive days, we took turns lying on the board, while flushing twenty gallons of purified water and herbs through our colons over a period of an hour and a half to two hours. Between the lemonade and

> Tom and Tamara arrived to see my father in poor shape and my sister suffering from insomnia, a severe case of Tourette's Syndrome, and anxiety. I was at the mercy of my temper with just a slightly better managed case of Tourette's. And Mom was pulling her hair out trying to deal with a family of nut jobs.
>
> **DAN WIONS**

the Colema Board, the things that oozed from our bodies could have inspired a bestselling series of sci-fi horror novels. I'll spare you the truly gory details, but suffice it to say that years of eating a typical American diet had resulted in a buildup of toxins and residual matter that had become a breeding ground for viruses, bacteria, and parasites. The objective of these procedures was to rest our digestive organs, reactivate our immune systems, and prevent further invitation to disease by eliminating this waste. To help repair the damage already done to our bodies, Tom and Tamara provided us with other therapies, plus what I refer to as "spiritual work."

Tom and Tamara were with us for only a couple of weeks. Their work opened up many opportunities, but also left us with many questions. By the time of their departure, we were far from expert on the foreign practices they had recommended. To help bridge the gap after their departure, they introduced us to their friend, Sue Lawton.

Describing the kind of work that Sue does defies simple explanation. She calls herself a "transition midwife." In this role, her primary focus (as I understand it) is helping people with terminal illnesses to orchestrate their departure with greater peace of mind, body, and spirit. One of the questions I always pose to a practitioner when I begin working with them is, "What experience have you had in treating people with ALS and with what results?" A response of "no experience" and/or "no positive results" is not always a deal breaker. But, since doctors claim there is no cure for ALS, knowing what background a practitioner is starting with is important to me.

Sue's answer to this question was at once startling and inspiring. While she had worked with several ALS patients, she told me that I was the first one who had made the choice to live. At first I was stunned. Reflecting on the many conversations I had had with others in my situation, I began to understand how this was possible, especially considering her occupation. People tend to seek her out when they have made a choice different from my own.

What I found inspiring was her further response about the possibilities. She didn't hesitate for a moment to affirm the potential for my full recovery. In her view, my will and my intention to recover were enough to secure success. Her perspective was both reassuring and motivating. Sue's work with me focused around the use of essential oils, affirmations (statements that you recite to keep your mind focused positively), and supplements. Through her support and influence, I explored the spiritual realm more deeply and broadly than I ever would have expected. This work has been a huge source of growth and perspective, contributing significantly to my efforts to live out my intention.

While my family and I experienced a good deal of excitement over the possibilities introduced to us by Tom, Tamara, and Sue, 2006 was a difficult year. The time between my last few updates had grown significantly longer than between earlier ones. This was a reflection of my increased loss of weight, strength, and energy from disease progression and the demands of QRA and the lemonade on my weakened body. By the end of 2006, my original 185-pound frame had diminished to a mere 99 pounds.

Another thing that made 2006 a tough year was the home-health-aide issue. It is no small thing to be forced by circumstances to invite a stranger home to help you with things like showering, peeing, and wiping your butt. Add to that the difficulty of finding an aide who is both willing and able to do all that's required, but who is also a good personality and temperament fit. Between April and December of '06, we went through five different aides, and had still not found the right one.

By the end of the year, having not communicated to my supporters since April, it was time to update them on the big changes that had occurred.

HEALTH UPDATE: 12/09/06

Sorry it's been so long since my last update. I have been waiting until I was able to report some dramatically positive changes. And while the hoped-for changes are taking longer than I would like, it occurred to me that many of you may be assuming that news about me would be negative since it has been so long since the last health update. My friend, Jim, is providing really crappy typing skills (his personal assessment, although one with which I concur) to help me get through this, but he can still do it faster than I can with my hunt-and-peck method using a mouse and an on-screen keyboard.

A lot has changed in my treatment plan. I am no longer trying to suck down 150 pills per day. Although continuing to see the same nutritionist, I am being more selective about which of her suggestions to employ. The problem is that the program had become much too time consuming. It was becoming the focus of my life, and it was getting depressing. Unaware of alternatives, I was afraid to stop. Her approach was not without benefits, but it was failing to deliver the desired degree of progress. Interestingly enough, Wendy (the nutritionist) herself came up with the next road in this incredible journey. She referred me to a Canadian couple who work with, among other things, an amazing detoxing program involving a special mixture of lemonade. Yes, that's right, I said lemonade. The purpose of the lemonade, a combination of freshly squeezed lemon juice, cayenne pepper, maple syrup, and purified water, is to allow the body to remove all kinds of toxins, largely by doing a thorough cleansing of the bowels, and by lightening the digestive load.

The lemonade, however, is only the tip of the iceberg for the total program. We also: went through ten days of colon cleansing; learned how to use essential oils; experienced Vitaflex therapy (a form of reflexology); had some massage work done; and learned how to do color therapy

(the use of colored lighting to treat the body
with subtle frequencies).

Last, but most importantly, we learned how to
shift our thinking in a very powerful, health-
affirming way. I learned through this experience
that, despite efforts to be positively focused,
many aspects of my thought process were literally
contributing to my demise. We began this process
at the end of July. Since then, I have alternated
between stints on the lemonade cleanse and periods
on solid food and supplements.

So, what difference has all this made? Well, I am
back to getting comments about how great I look,
but beyond that there have also been benefits in
my breathing and hand strength. These are
fluctuating benefits, however, since my body is
currently using a lot of energy to rebuild. This
is according to the most recent practitioner in my
life, Sue Lawton, who is a nurse, a psychologist,
and a psychic (there goes that "woo-woo" stuff
again). Sue has been very helpful in teaching me
how to use the oils and how to remain positively
focused using affirmations.

My breathing remains in the low 20-percent range,
but anything other than a reduction in capacity is
great news! During my current period on solid
food, I have managed to gain SIX pounds in the
last six weeks! My current health aide has some
special skills as a martial arts trainer, which he
is using to help me maintain mobility and recover
muscle strength. With his help, I am expecting
that the pounds will be converted into muscle. The
days have been more enjoyable and more productive,

and I am closer to feeling convinced that I am on the road to recovery.

Again, knowing that you guys are out there caring and praying for me also continues to be a big part of what keeps me going. Thanks, as always, for being there. By the way, those of you looking for evidence of Jim's crappy typing, I can only say thank heaven for spell check.

Joe

CHAPTER TEN

Nonsensical New Age

Growth and Enlightenment

As a consultant who'd spent 30 years coaching big time executives, Dad had a bit of a pride hurdle to jump over. Tom, while maybe a little arrogant, was a calm and patient man. He took Dad through a visualization exercise that addressed issues around his mother, forgiveness, security, and fear. It was a defining moment that ended in a huge emotional release, and enabled Dad to step back and admit: "OK, if I knew this stuff already, I might not be sitting in this wheelchair." This one shift in mindset had a more drastic impact on his condition than any treatments prior to that day.

DAN WIONS

The work that began with Tom, Tamara, and Sue opened up possibilities for healing that I would never have thought to explore—what I will refer to loosely as "spiritual healing." It is through these types of practices that I have achieved the most success in combating ALS. I use the term "spiritual" not so much in a religious sense—although it can include religious belief and practice—but rather in reference to activities that attract and direct the flow of positive healing energy. Tom and Tamara taught me that the human brain operates like a simple but very powerful computer. If you put positive information into it, it acts on that information and sends out positive signals to the body. Conversely, if you think negative thoughts, the brain sends out negative signals to the body.

For example, if your hand is paralyzed and you accept this condition as permanent, the brain sends the messages through the nervous system that your hand cannot and will not move. If, however, you envision your hand in motion and continually reaffirm your intention to move it, your brain will send the messages necessary to repair the damage, eventually enabling the hand to move. Put more simply, if you put positive energy out, good things happen. If you put negative energy out, bad things happen.

In the video seminar, *The Secret*, this process is explained as a law of quantum physics called the "Law of Attraction." Morris Goodman, who appears in the film, used the Law of Attraction to regain his total mobility against all odds. Following a plane crash in which he sustained severe spinal cord damage, doctors told him that the opening and closing of his eyelids was the only physical movement of which he would be capable for the rest of his life. Convinced of his ability to heal, despite the doctors' prognosis, Goodman confronted this nightmare with a positive determination. Achieving complete recovery of his physical capacities within a year and a half, he became known as "The Miracle Man."

My ongoing education in applying the Law of Attraction and other spiritual healing approaches has quite literally saved my life. When one thinks of a turning point in the course of a life-threatening illness, what probably comes most quickly to mind are physical changes in health. For me, the turning point in my journey with ALS was much more subtle. It began with the incredible shift in mind-set that occurred through my work with Tom and Tamara.

Who would have imagined I was thinking myself to death or that I could think myself to recovery? Here I was taking pride in my strength and positive attitude, never suspecting that, on a daily basis, I was subtly undermining my intention to recover with those very thoughts. The shift in thinking that Tom and Tamara helped me to achieve and the resources to which they exposed me opened up whole new ways for me to see myself, others, and the world. At the risk of sounding like a religious fanatic, it was almost like being reborn. I read Louise Hay's, *You Can Heal Your Life*, and learned to replace my fears and worries with affirmations. And when I first watched the movie, *The Secret*, at their urging, I began learning how to use The Law of Attraction to draw positive energy and the things I want in life toward me, instead of attracting the opposite by worrying about the negative possibilities.

From this beginning, I discovered that the key to my survival and recovery lay less in treating my body than in treating my brain and my heart. Suddenly the pipeline of possible treatments that had seemed so dry before Tom and Tamara's arrival was flowing with a rush of options. Six months after their visit, I was using "The Healing Codes" (a process using prayers, intentions, and a series of hand positions directing energy to several healing zones around the head and face) to surface and resolve "cellular memories" that had been driving the dysfunctional thoughts and behaviors contributing to my illness. A year later, I discovered *The Journey*, by Brandon Bays, and found a practitioner to help me apply her approach. Practicing Brandon's processes of physical and emotional journeys helped me to accelerate the kind of progress I had been making with The Healing Codes. You may be wondering just what kind of progress that was.

As an example, the aches and pains that had been progressively intensifying as my body weakened miraculously disappeared. My body became more relaxed and easier to move within the range of motion that I still had. My energy level increased dramatically. There were even measurable improvements in my breathing capacity.

Despite my openness to trying whatever might work, my perception of many of these practices initially suffered from what I think of as the "Woo Woo Factor." Like most people, I exercise some skepticism about practices with which I am unfamiliar. Some of these practices were so far outside my experience and knowledge base that they seemed almost too absurd to seriously consider. Had I not been coming from a place where the trusted paradigm (i.e., traditional Western medicine) offered no desirable options, I might not have been open to travel these alternative and spiritual paths. The results speak for themselves. This book would probably never have been written had I not taken this route.

HEALTH UPDATE: 4/29/07

While I'm not yet running laps around the block, I continue to take small steps in the right direction. My protocol continues to evolve. What hasn't changed since the last time I wrote is my focus on gratitude and affirmations. I am taking a few more daily supplements, but the total number of capsules is under twenty—a far cry from the pint of pills I was swallowing every day last summer. I also continue to use the lemonade cleanse every two to three months and the essential oils and color therapy periodically as well. Additions to the process include the use of a modality known as "The Healing Codes." These are, in a way, an extension of the affirmation process. If you want to learn more, you can consult the website, *www.thehealingcodes.com*. I am also beginning to use a form of sound therapy through a meditation program called Sonic Access, which I just began.

On the results side of the equation, I continue to see subtle evidence that my body is rebuilding itself. While these indicators come and go, periodic improvements in my breathing and hand-and-arm strength continue to convince me that I'm on the right track. As time passes, I grow less and less concerned that when my breathing or strength decreases it may be due to progression of the disease. The evidence that this is not the case lies in the fact that they continue to come back. This suggests that the lapses are more likely a result of my body needing to use its energy for rebuilding, which takes strength away from other functions. I am also continuing to hold and even gain weight between cleanses. A few weeks ago, I was back up to the 108 pounds that I weighed before my last cleanse in January. I suspect I've gained a few pounds since then as well.

The most impressive changes that have occurred seem to be stemming from my use of The Healing Codes, which began in February. By tapping into deeply held cellular memories, I have been unearthing unconscious beliefs that I am convinced have not only caused this disease but have also blocked my efforts to recover. As I peel away the layers, I grow more and more certain that I am getting closer to a dramatic turning point in my condition.

Joe

The more I applied these spiritual techniques, the more attractive they became. Finally, I had found something that was making a concrete and sustainable difference in the way I was feeling and functioning. I became highly motivated to continue exploring this path.

HEALTH UPDATE: 9/25/07

As I said in the last update, I'm still not running laps around the block. However, I am putting a lot more miles on my wheelchair of late. A number of changes this summer have positively impacted my health and quality of life. So, I thought this might be a good time to update you on some of the highlights.

A focus on gratitude, affirmations, meditation, and The Healing Codes continues to be at the core of my protocol. Currently, I am taking no supplements at all. Although that may change from time to time, the plan is to keep my pill intake limited to about twenty per day. In May, I completed my fifth lemonade cleanse since July '06, reaching the goal of 100 days of cleansing

within the first year. I will continue with the
lemonade cleanse periodically, but right now the
cost of lemons is prohibitive (it can take almost
an entire crate of lemons to do a 10-day cleanse).
More importantly, I think weight gain is a bigger
priority than further intensive cleansing at the
moment. By the end of my last cleanse in May, I
had dropped back to 106 pounds. It took me until
the end of August to get back to the 113 pounds
that I weighed before the cleanse, which
represents my highest weight since the low of 99
pounds last winter. Essential oils and color
therapy also continue to be part of my program,
but on a limited and selective basis.

The latest addition to my protocol is yet another
change in diet. I am currently eating primarily
raw vegetables and fruits in salad and juice form.
It is actually quite tasty and filling and holds
huge promise for rebuilding my body. After only a
month, I have already experienced benefits in
energy and endurance.

So, you're probably wondering, "What difference
has all this made?" Well, as a result of the
increased energy and endurance, Diane and I have
been able to take more frequent and longer walks
than I was capable of even this past spring. On
several occasions, I was able to keep my
wheelchair going for two miles or more without a
stop. This is about a fourfold improvement. My
breathing seems to be slowly improving, allowing
me longer periods of time without use of the Bi-
PAP. I can actually see my diaphragm moving in the
right direction now and, when not on the Bi-PAP, I
am able to breathe without excessive use of my

chest muscles. My color has improved so much that people keep commenting on how good I look. Now I can *totally* get rid of all my cosmetic products!!! In all seriousness, we recently compared my current appearance with a picture that was taken of me last December. The degree of improvement was startling. Last but not least, my bodily functions have grown much more reliable, enabling me to get out of the house more frequently.

Diane and I have been able to get out to restaurants, go shopping together, and visit friends. We've managed about a dozen outings since the spring. This past weekend, I made it to all three Yom Kippur services (Friday night, Saturday morning and evening) for the first time in about three years. Capping off the weekend, we attended the induction of a close friend's son into the Eagle Scouts, followed by a celebratory barbecue. That's four outings over three days! I can't tell you how much that adds to my confidence that full recovery is in my future.

Joe

CHAPTER ELEVEN

Guidance From the Gut

One area that I thought I had under control was diet. For most of the ten years or so preceding my diagnosis, my diet had been largely vegan. Between my eating habits and my exercise regimen, I was pretty well convinced that I was doing what was needed to stay healthy. This made my diagnosis that much more of a shock. From 2002, when my pursuit of alternative medical treatment began, until 2007, when I moved to a new level, I had received varying dietary recommendations from nearly every practitioner I worked with. It wasn't until the summer of 2007 that I truly began to understand the impact that diet can have on physical, emotional, and psychological health.

Knowledge gained that summer led me to shift my diet exclusively to raw fruits and vegetables, as mentioned briefly in my 9/25/07 Health Update. The person who brought me to the doorstep of this new level of learning was none other than my own son, Dan. Both of my children had developed some healthy lifestyle practices, especially in the area of exercise. Dan, however, developed an extraordinarily intense focus on health issues, particularly in the area of diet. He is quite aware of how I have chosen to live my life, and I think my wife and I can fairly take some of the credit for having influenced his attention to diet and exercise. Knowing that I had always gone to great lengths to take care of myself and yet had still contracted one of the most devastating diseases known to man fed his motivation to learn more and more about proper fuel and human body care. By the age of 29, after two years of intensive research, Dan had become our family's resident guru on building health through diet.

His significant influence on my eating behavior began with his early investigations of a raw vegan diet in that summer of 2007. That is when he introduced me to *The Vegetarian Guide to Diet and Salad*, by

Dr. Norman Walker. Coming from a mostly vegetarian diet, a raw fruit and vegetable diet was certainly less of a leap than it would be for most people. Still, I must admit to some strong initial skepticism that this seemingly extreme step was justifiable. As I read Walker's book, I became more and more intrigued by his explanation of how the human body builds and replaces cells to maintain health. Following is a brief explanation of Walker's work. I encourage you to read his short and easily "digestible" book (sorry, I couldn't resist) for yourself to get a completely accurate picture of what he has to offer.

Walker explains, in fairly simple language, how the body uses enzymes to construct the amino acid chains that it needs to build and replace healthy cells. He further explains that the purest and most potent source of enzymes is found in raw fruits and vegetables. Cooking destroys or damages the enzymes, vitamins, and minerals found in food, to the point where much of the nutritional value becomes compromised, or totally lost, depending on the type of food and cooking method. We compound the problem when we eat large quantities of animal-based foods, especially when our digestive and immune systems are already compromised, since the proteins available from these sources are not readily bio-available. Thus, the body must first expend energy to break down these foods into enzymes, which must then be reassembled into amino acid chains that the body can use. Not only is additional energy required to

> When I was a junior in high school, our whole family experimented with a vegan diet. Dad stayed with it long after the rest of us succumbed to our cravings for bagels and lox, pizza, ice cream, and hamburgers. Even with that year-long experiment, however, we still had no clue what we were doing, nor did we have any exposure to the world of healthful cleansing and fasting, outside of barely making it through a Yom Kippur day fast once a year.
>
> Tom, Tamara, and Dr. Graham opened our eyes to what it meant to reset and nourish the body. Additionally, they showed us how that process removed our cravings altogether. We learned that one can be vegan simply by omitting animal products, but being vegan didn't necessarily have anything to do with being healthy. Our diet had included highly processed foods like potato chips, white flour, corn syrup, and vegetable oils. They also happen to be a recipe for disease.
>
> **DAN WIONS**

accomplish this, but the subsequent product (again, compromised by cooking) is far inferior to what we get when we eat fresh fruits and vegetables in their natural state. This is one of the reasons why, Walker contends, the typical American diet will normally sustain the human body for about forty to fifty years, at which point many people begin to contract serious illnesses or lose their physical vibrancy. After that, the body simply begins to break down from malnutrition.

Walker also advocates juicing. His rationale is that we cannot consume enough raw fruit and vegetables to satisfy our body's needs for fresh enzymes. He offers significant guidance on the relative potency of a wide variety of fruits and vegetables, and even offers a list of approximately seventy different salad recipes in this little book. I am told that he lived on this diet in near-perfect health to the age of 107, at which point he died of accidental causes. Learning all of this made it easier to comply with my son's wishes and give it a try.

Within the first two weeks, I experienced a surge in energy like nothing I had gotten from any previous treatment. The best example was the change in the strength of my right hand, which I use to operate the driving stick of my wheelchair. Prior to starting Walker's diet, I had been capable of holding the stick in place for the three-quarter-mile "walk" around the block that I enjoy with my wife, but I would have to stop three or four times to adjust my hand position or rest. Within two weeks, though, the walks had stretched to three and a half miles, with no more than one or two stops. I was sold on raw vegan as the way to go.

Dan's general approach was to research regimens that allowed for a maximum amount of balanced nutrients, while taking into account rules of food combining and minimizing digestive effort. It is not a huge surprise that this translated into mostly uncooked fruits and vegetables. Many variations exist on the raw, or mostly raw, vegan diet, each with its own set of passionate followers and promoters. My son and I researched and experimented with many of these variations to find what worked for us.

By the time I had become entrenched in my new diet plan, Dan had already moved to another book by a doctor and exercise physiologist who coached a number of the world's leading athletes and even some movie stars on how to adjust their diet and exercise to achieve optimal results. Unlike Walker, Dr. Graham does not believe juicing is necessary, but instead recommends whole fruits, and lots of them at once, much like foraging primates (or children who have found a tree). He also advocates supplementing the fruits in these mono-meals with abundant quantities of leafy green vegetables. Unlike Walker, Graham also places an emphasis on minimizing fat in the diet. He offers some very compelling research evidence to support the capacity of his diet to promote optimal health and avoid serious illness.

This is just a glimpse of the work of these two men through my eyes. The purpose of including this information here is to highlight the fact that dietary changes had as big an impact on stabilizing and/or improving my condition as anything I had tried to date. Since shifting my diet toward a low fat raw vegan approach, I have experienced improvements in my energy, skin color, sleep patterns, and more. I continue to be extremely optimistic about the prospects for further improvements.

HEALTH UPDATE: 1/12/08

Happy New Year!

While physical changes continue to elude me, things for the most part continue to go well. I have lost a tiny bit more function in my hands and arms, but it has not made any appreciable difference in my lifestyle. I can still brush my teeth after the toothbrush is inserted in my mouth—by moving the brush head with my tongue, lips and head movement while trapping the barrel between my overlapped hands on the edge of the countertop. My breathing has also remained fairly stable for the past year, and I continue to get out of the house more often.

The treatment plan has changed only slightly since the last update in September. I continue to focus on gratitude, affirmations, meditation, The Healing Codes, and the raw fruit and vegetable diet. I have also been functioning without the help of any supplements now for several months. Additions to my regimen include some modifications to diet, an increased emphasis on exercise, and a resumption of acupuncture treatments.

The dietary changes involve a reduction of juicing and a focus on "mono-meals." Mono-meals simply mean I am eating meals with greater quantities of individual fruits and vegetables with less variety at each meal. A typical lunch might be four or five large leaves of romaine lettuce with five apples, or six bananas, or three mangoes. The idea is to take in enough of each item to get the full nutritional value that it has to offer. These ideas come from the work of Dr. Douglas Graham, author of *The 80/10/10 Diet*. I am currently working with him through e-mails, and am evolving a customized diet and exercise plan to optimize healing. Stay tuned—this should be interesting.

Back in September, I resumed acupuncture treatments with Dr. Xie in Princeton. Some of you may recall that after working with her for several months about three years ago, while still under the care of Dr. Kessler in Germany, and also using Bu Nao Gao (BNG), we stopped, sensing there was some kind of energy blockage that was impeding the accumulation of energy from her treatments. As you know, I have since done a great deal of physical, emotional, and spiritual cleansing, and Dr. Xie agreed that the time might be right to give acupuncture another try. Since resuming this treatment, my energy levels have consistently increased. While this has not yet translated into physical function, Dr. Xie is confident that it will over time, as she has had some success with related diagnoses. It could take a year before results are evident, but after almost eight years of living with this disease, a year really doesn't seem that long.

My weight has been a little up and down with the ongoing experimentation in diet, ranging from about 112 to 119 pounds. This is in contrast to my low point a year ago of 99 pounds, but hopefully, the new diet and exercise program will help build more muscle weight as opposed to just fat. About every six months, the hospice nurse measures the circumference of my arms and legs. Last week, we discovered gains in each thigh of a centimeter or more and smaller improvements in my forearms. This additional mass bodes well for the development of muscle tissue as opposed to just adding weight around my waist.

Although spending several hours a day at the computer, it is still difficult to type any lengthy e-mails (today's health update, by the way, comes to you courtesy of June Halper's nimble fingers). The fact that I am able to move my computer mouse around in my lap for several hours a day reflects the energy level that the current regimen is yielding. With the help of a hospice volunteer, I am also making some significant progress on a book about my experiences with ALS (I'll expect all of you to buy several copies and encourage others to buy it as well. Great retirement plan, huh?)

That pretty much sums up how I'm doing. I hope
2008 is off to a great start for you and that it
yields lots of love, health, happiness, and
prosperity. Thanks, as always, for being there,
for caring, and for contributing to the positive
life force that keeps me going.

Joe

There have been few instances in which I have resumed a particular treatment once I had decided to move on from it. Acupuncture, as you read in the 1/12/08 Health Update, is one of them. There are several reasons for my decision to resume this treatment. One is that Dr. Xie's modest past successes with patients having similar diagnoses is encouraging and intriguing. Another is that acupuncture has to do with the channeling and strengthening of energy flow, which links it to what I have been referring to as "spiritual" modalities. Practices like affirmations, The Law of Attraction, The Healing Codes, and the Journey, all, at least in part, involve a refocusing of the mind. Part of my healing process has been to learn to accept the notion that the mind's physical entity, the brain, is essentially an organic machine designed to generate and receive electronic messages, but within these messages, a connection emerges. As a means of encouraging a more positive flow of the electrical energy of the brain, these "spiritual" practices have something in common with acupuncture. The fact that these approaches have rendered some of my best results to date further strengthens my confidence that acupuncture can be effective in restoring some mobility.

Finally, there is my personal experience with this modality. After a treatment I feel greater strength in my hands and more energy overall. This, combined with the doctor's assessment that the energy keeps building in my system, has led me to anticipate further improvements over time. I hope the strength and energy gained from my diet will keep me steady until these additional benefits are realized.

HEALTH UPDATE: 4/26/08

This update starts with a mildly sour note for a
very simple reason: I don't have much bad news to
report! I might as well get it out of the way
early: the loss of hand strength reported in
January has not yet reversed.

That's it!

This translates into continued difficulty in
operating the adjustment buttons on my wheel
chair. While it is somewhat disappointing, this
inconvenience pales in comparison to the positive
changes that I have experienced since the last
update.

Have I created enough anticipation yet, or shall I
continue to build the suspense a little longer?
No? OK, so here is the good news: above the weak
fingers, the arms seem a little stronger and have
a slightly greater range of motion. Brushing my
teeth has become much easier. I am now able to
complete the task nonstop almost every time, and
with only a fraction of the energy it used to
take. My weight is now up to 121 lbs., my neck and
abdominal muscles feel a little stronger, and
there seems to be a tiny bit more movement in my
legs. Most important of all, my breathing capacity
has reached consecutive two-year highs for the
past three months!

The treatment plan remains relatively unchanged
since January, with continued focus on gratitude,
affirmations, meditation, The Healing Codes, and
the 80/10/10 diet. I continue to evolve my
exercise program and go for acupuncture treatments
on a weekly basis. The only significant changes

since last time have been the addition of another mind/body/spiritual type practice, called "Journeying," and some additional bodywork on my ribs to assist in breathing. The Journey process, like The Healing Codes, is a mechanism for clearing cellular memories that can contribute to illness. I learned about it in a book by Brandon Bays called, (are you ready?) *The Journey*. I highly recommend the book—it is a great read and a fascinating process. I hired a practitioner at the beginning of April to take me through it for several hours. It was intense, exhausting, and extremely productive. I am able to draw on elements of the experience daily and am convinced that this process has played a significant role in recent improvements.

As in January, lengthy e-mails continue to be a challenge. Today's health update, by the way, comes to you through my friend Hongbo's nimble fingers. Progress on the book has accelerated, and if all goes well it should be completed this year. So, get those checkbooks and credit cards ready!

Diane is enjoying a few well-deserved days of rest during her spring break before launching into the last rush of spring concerts, including the big one on May 7. Dan has been running himself ragged playing in concerts from New Brunswick to Allentown, PA to Philadelphia to Wilmington, DE. He is tired but looking forward to the paychecks. Julie is about two weeks away from completing her associate's degree at Raritan Valley Community College and is praying for the scriptwriters to complete their work so that Spike Lee can finally shoot the movie she won a lead in last summer.

That pretty much sums up how we're doing. We are looking forward to the next SerenAide benefit concert that Diane's students have been coordinating for us for the past four years. That will be happening on Wednesday, May 28, at 7 p.m., at J.P. Stevens High School in Edison. The first year of this concert was a tear-jerking, heart-warming expression of love for an extraordinary teacher (my wife), by her students. While the concert continues to be a very moving tribute to Diane, it has also evolved into a fairly polished and entertaining evening of music. Please join us if you can. We'd love to share the experience with you.

> Mrs. Wions has been my inspiration for my entire life. She has shaped my personality and my life philosophy, and she gave me a second family. Mr. Wions is one of the most inspiring people I have ever met. He faced every day, every ounce of suffering, with an optimistic outlook and a smile on his face. SerenAIDe really builds love, and love flourishes. Seeing direct and positive results on Mr. and Mrs. Wions made me realize that a group of students can make such a difference. I am still surprised at this power.
>
> **AMY KIM**
> J.P. STEVENS CHOIR
> ALUMNA

I hope your world is wonderful. Thanks, as always, for being part of mine, for caring, and for contributing to the positive life force that keeps me going.

Joe

Something that had become very clear by this time was that the best input on how to manage my health was no longer coming from practitioners, but from my own body. I was becoming more and more focused on how I felt and functioned in relation to the various practices and treatments. At this point in the search, my spiritual regimen, dietary practices, exercise, and acupuncture seemed to be keeping me at least stable and perhaps improving. While my ability to push the control buttons on the wheelchair had diminished, the ability to hold onto and manage a toothbrush had improved. My skin was in excellent shape, bodily functions were behaving consistently, sleep interruptions were on the decline, and there were even signs that my breathing was improving.

One of the many people who contributed to my well-being on a regular basis was a man named Nick Klevans. Nick is a kind of mind/bodywork therapist who practices something called "integrative therapy," and volunteers his time through hospice. In addition to inflicting a great deal of therapeutic pain—which he seemed to enjoy far too much—Nick also provided regular feedback on how my body was functioning energetically. He often expressed amazement at how well it was working, given the level of paralysis. With almost every bi-monthly visit, he would tease me, "You are the healthiest sick person I know."

As a video biographer, I've found a calling in capturing people's life stories to save for posterity and to pass on to future generations. My inspiration toward this calling came from none other than Joe, who was one of my hospice patients for 5 years. I would come to his home every couple of weeks to do some bodywork on him and to engage in the type of deep philosophical conversations we both enjoyed. On one such visit, I asked him if I could film his life story. At the time, I didn't even own a video camera. Joe has become a "guiding angel" in my mission to encourage people to get their life stories documented, regardless of their age or state of health.

NICK KLEVANS
HOSPICE VOLUNTEER, FRIEND

CHAPTER TWELVE

Search for Complete Healing

With the writing of each health update, I would reflect deeply on what had changed since my last communiqué. The unevenness of developments in my physical status could make it very difficult to articulate the gains. I wanted so desperately to convince myself and my readers that the improvements were real, but unless the changes were truly dramatic, I couldn't effectively describe my progress. There were times when this struggle produced long delays in getting out the next update.

HEALTH UPDATE: 12/13/08

I can't believe it has been almost eight months since my last update. I am guessing that the long delay has left some of you concerned about my health and others relieved at having less reading to do. So, regardless of which camp you fall into, please accept my apologies.

The first piece of news is obvious, given your receipt of this e-mail: I am still here! While my hands are working no better, they are no weaker, and I am still able to work my toothbrush as effectively as described in the April update. Although there have been some ups and downs, my weight has held at about 120 lbs. Similarly, breathing capacity has fluctuated, but it is currently holding in a range of about 1.4 to 1.7 liters. This is roughly 20-25 percent of normal capacity.

Treatment efforts this year have focused primarily on diet, detoxing, and spiritual/attitude/energy practices. Gratitude, affirmations, meditation, The Healing Codes, and the 80/10/10 diet continue to be core parts of my program. I also continue to evolve the exercise regimen and go for acupuncture treatments on a weekly basis. Recently, I have intensified my work with the Journey process and employed the efforts of a healer who works with me daily over the phone. José, the healer, believes he is making progress in eliminating free radicals and toxins and improving the communication between my muscles, nerves and more. His work has yet to translate into many sustained, tangible changes in my ability to move and function, but I am hopeful that it will in time. One of the clear indicators of the potential in his work is the expansion of airflow in my left lung, which was noted by both my respiratory therapist and my hospice nurse.

I visited Joe a few times over the years, and he stayed with us in California. I had been following his emails for years as his mobility crept away, so when I visited in 2008, I was prepared to see him in a wheelchair.

What I was not expecting was how perfectly healthy he appeared to be inside of his battered body. Joe was still Joe, but in much sharper detail: a strong will, a smart mouth, and a can-do attitude that carries everyone along. The hands that fed him (a lettuce smoothie...um, YUM?) were not his own, but he showed me how he wrote his emails using someone's brilliant invention: a typing pad attached to his wheelchair. Joe seems to have transferred all the power his body lost into his wonderful writing.

I am already imagining the next time we meet. I fully expect him to be on his feet in front of a crowd, showing people everywhere what we all want to believe is true: that with hard work and in the right spirit, "impossible" is just another word to laugh at.

KRISTEN CAVEN

Because lengthy e-mails continue to be a challenge, today's health update again comes to you through the fingers of Hongbo. (Thank you Hongbo's fingers!). The first draft of my book seems to be complete, and revisions are in progress.

Diane just polished off another outstanding winter concert and is already preparing her students for the spring concert series. Dan continues to burn the candle at both ends, playing in concerts from Hartford to Washington DC to Switzerland to Mexico. He is tired but enjoying an increasing quality of musical engagements and is happy to get paid for what he loves to do. He is also continuing to make progress in building his Live Music Consulting business, which you can read about at www.livemusicconsulting.com. Julie completed her degree back in May and, since then, has started her own business selling her artwork in the form of note cards. You can view her work at *www.creationsbyjulie.net*. She is also working furiously, doing substitute teaching, babysitting, and catering work, trying to save up enough money to bankroll a move back into New York City to continue pursuit of her acting and modeling career. The movie that she was cast in died and has been revived. We are still hoping they will actually shoot the thing someday, but Julie is not sitting around waiting for that to happen.

That pretty much sums up how we're doing. Let me take this opportunity to wish you a wonderful holiday season and a bright new year.

Joe

So the road to recovery had proven to be a bumpy one. This should come as no surprise, given that my quest for full recovery totally defied conventional medical wisdom. While the key to regaining more strength and movement in the arms and legs continued to elude me, my resolve was buoyed by continued improvements in overall health. I continued to explore new treatments and marvel at the strength acquired from the physical, emotional, mental and spiritual growth achieved to date. These gains helped me to deal with life's unexpected adventures with more balance and poise than would have been possible in the past.

HEALTH UPDATE: 4/18/09

I hope your 2009 has been off to a good start. Ours has been good for the most part, with some exciting adventures along the way. The first excitement came during the last week in January. This was when the Philadelphia chapter of the ALS Association called to tell me that, due to budget cutbacks, they would no longer be able to subsidize the costs for my live-in health aide. Considering that we couldn't afford the agency fees we were paying without the ALSA support, and that function without the help of an aide is currently not an option, this news was a pretty serious attention-grabber. As if that weren't exciting enough, they were only giving me five days' notice!

Fortunately, they agreed to grant me an extension to the end of February, so I could figure out how to deal with the situation. My care manager, Bonnie Kramer, and I both got busy on the phone looking for private aides and non-state-certified agencies that might be able to provide less expensive care. We found success with an agency that places aides who come mostly from Russia and Eastern Europe. Gintaras (Jimmy) Franka, who hails from Lithuania, has now been working with me for about two months. The silver lining in all this is that Jimmy has turned out to be the best live-in help I have ever had. We are hoping he will be staying with us for as long as we need him.

Another adventure occurred a few weeks ago during a visit to the health food store in Princeton when my Bi-PAP (breathing machine) failed. We quickly returned to the van, but couldn't get it working there either, and I felt myself fading. We called Diane to bring the spare Bi-PAP, but she was thirty minutes away. The next call was 911.

The first responders arrived quickly and behaved compassionately but, regrettably, failed to do the most important thing: listen to the patient. They strapped on an oxygen mask, which made it even more difficult to project my voice as my diaphragm became increasingly overtaxed and my air supply continued to fade. When I regained consciousness in the emergency room, the first faces I saw were Dan's, then Julie's, and then Diane's. They had hooked me up to the extra Bi-PAP, and I was coming around. Unfortunately, by the time my family arrived, the medical staff had already inserted IVs in both wrists, sliced my clothes to shreds, and plastered thirty or forty electrodes to my torso.

Thankfully, Diane was able to successfully intervene and prevent further unnecessary testing and procedures. After an hour on the Bi-PAP and a few gulps of apple juice, I was good to go home.

Lessons learned: Don't travel without back-up equipment, and order a medical alert tag with breathing support instructions! Hopefully, future lessons will be born of less exciting circumstances.

One very positive outcome of both of these experiences is that each created a heightened awareness of the degree to which my spiritual growth has helped in dealing with difficult situations. In both instances, I found myself, after only a few brief moments of panic, focusing my attention on the present moment and quickly launching into appropriate action, instead of wasting energy on worries about what could go wrong. I stayed focused and relaxed, and took care of business. That common aspect of my adventures felt very, very good.

As far as physical function is concerned, there are no dramatic changes to report, but there are some interesting developments. My hands are working about the same, although working on the computer tires them out more quickly. An adjustment at the bathroom sink has made the chore of brushing my teeth considerably easier. We now use a folded towel on the edge of the vanity to prop up my hands. This brings the toothbrush closer to my mouth, thereby reducing the strain on my neck, back, and abdominal muscles. In addition, the towel slides across the sink counter surface much more easily than my sweaty palms. The net result is greater and easier mobility moving the toothbrush with far less exhaustion.

My weight continues to hold at about 120 lbs., give or take a few in any given month. I prefer to keep it there until some of it starts turning into muscle weight. There is currently more belly than I care to see. The doctors, of course, would claim that loss of muscle tissue with ALS is irreversible. But, if I believed everything the doctors say, I'd be pushing up daisies by now. It's hard to believe I've been living with the symptoms of this illness for nine years. May 9 will mark the sixth anniversary of the confirmed diagnosis. That means I've already beaten the odds by one to four years, depending on how you calculate it.

Breathing capacity measures provide the most promising news. In December, I was fairly excited to report that it had gotten back up to as high as 1.7 liters. Since then, the numbers have continued to increase, and yesterday it hit 2.85 liters. That's the best it's been in three years! The trick now is to find a way to increase the strength and endurance of my diaphragm, in order to take advantage of the increased capacity and spend longer periods of time off the Bi-PAP.

One new addition to my regimen of gratitude, affirmations, meditation, a raw vegan diet, regular exercise, and acupuncture is in the area of detoxing. My Healing Codes coach recommended a substance called Miracle Mineral Supplement (MMS). MMS is a very simple solution of sodium chlorite that, when mixed with citric acid, becomes chlorine dioxide. Ingestion of this substance creates an explosion of oxygenation into the bloodstream. The oxygen molecules attach to and eliminate most known pathogens. Jim Humble, the developer of MMS, has tracked its use in thousands of people with some amazing results. There have been reports of success in eliminating a wide variety of viruses, bacteria, toxins, and fungi.

I have also begun to use a supplement called Stem/Enhance, which is supposed to increase the body's stem cell production by as much as 30 to 40 percent. The hope is that to whatever degree ALS is caused by viral infection, MMS will clean it up sufficiently to give the increased presence of stem cells a chance to repair nerve damage. It's an encouraging theory. We'll see what happens.

My work with José Gonzales, the healer, also continues on a daily basis. José frequently cites progress in eliminating free radicals and toxins and in improving the communication between my muscles and nerves. He also continually finds new issues to address. The results of his work on my functioning to date include improved air flow in both lungs, reduction of problems with itching in some rather delicate areas, and fewer problems with food going down the wrong pipe.

'José the healer,' as we affectionately referred to him, was a shining example of the many people who came into our life the minute Dad began applying strategies like The Law of Attraction. After an initial examination in person, José spent time on the phone/Skype working on Dad in the morning, evening, and sometimes the middle of the day for years. During times when Dad was barely conscious, experiencing an adverse reaction to a supplement, or a detoxing symptom, a phone session with José would begin to revive him within seconds. Whether it was José's efforts or the power of placebo, it doesn't matter much to us. During the 5 or so years that José worked with Dad, he never took a dime from us. According to José, working with Dad helped him to evolve as a healer, allowing him to save countless other patients.

DAN WIONS

I still spend a good deal of time on the computer each day but need to take occasional breaks to give my hands and forearms a chance to regain their strength. My friend, Joan, was with me a few days ago to help with work on the book, so I also roped her into helping out with the typing of this health update. (Thanks, Joan!)

Diane is working her buns off preparing for the spring concert series. Next week, she gets on a plane with 180 of her choir members and a small army of dedicated parents and other chaperones to perform at Epcot Center in Florida. Dan ran a very successful marketing effort for Live Music Consulting at his first bridal show in January—hopefully, it will pay off big for him going into next year. Until then, he is running all over the place as usual, performing in orchestras and teaching horn. Julie is working hard at trying to complete the upgrading of her website so that stores and individuals can purchase her cards from it directly. Meanwhile, she continues to pay her bills by substitute teaching.

We are all looking forward to yet another SerenAide ALS benefit concert. It's hard to believe that Diane's students have now been coordinating this wonderful event for us for the past five years. The participants continue to honor Diane, and the performances just keep getting better and better.

That pretty much sums up how we're doing. Thanks, as always, for being there, for caring, and for being so consistently supportive.

Joe

One of the best outcomes of my progress to date was the degree of stability achieved that enabled me to continue the search with confidence and a sense of security about the future. Gone were the feelings of hopelessness and desperation with which this journey began. I rarely doubted the inevitability of success, and lived in constant awe of the blessings, gifts and insights I have acquired along the way

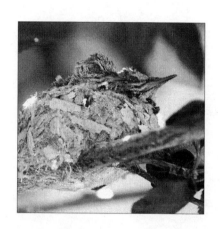

Part III

Blessings,
Gifts and
Insights

CHAPTER THIRTEEN

They Just Keep on Showing Up

As I mentioned in the introduction, it sounds and feels very strange to think of a devastating illness as a gift. Yet, while I am not happy to have contracted ALS, the learning it has brought and the continuous stream of blessings constantly amaze me. One of the most incredible of these blessings is the seemingly endless flow of people who keep streaming through my life to support my efforts to overcome this illness.

In addition to a very caring and engaged extended family, my wife and I are extremely fortunate to have several very close friends whose lives have been intertwined with ours for a very long time. We have always been there for each other through thick and thin. So, it was no surprise that our close friends and family showed up big time with their love and support when they heard about the diagnosis.

Over the several years that I have been living with ALS, however, many other people that I never would have imagined have come into our lives with acts of kindness and generosity. They have come with food. They have come to help with laundry and other household chores. They have come to do home maintenance and repairs and yard work. They have contributed money and run fundraising events to help pay medical expenses. Some have even helped with personal care when we had difficulty finding health aides. It has been an incredible display of the awesome depth of goodness of which human beings are capable. I feel truly blessed that we have been the recipients of this ongoing miracle.

Yet, I can't help but wonder what keeps fueling this endless display of altruism. What keeps drawing them here, to us, to me? For those who come to help my wife, there is no mystery involved. Diane is a wonderfully warm and supportive person who exudes an

143

When challenges surface, it can be a struggle to avoid harboring some level of resentment toward family and friends who cannot be there for you in the same capacity you have been, or would be, there for them. This resentment generally causes more harm to the person feeling it than it does to the person who triggered it. Every member of our family has faced this struggle at one time or another. Learning to accept people's limitations, to establish more realistic expectations, and to communicate our boundaries more effectively, are just some of the life skills this predicament brought to our awareness. In this chapter, Dad talks a lot about gratitude and describes interactions between himself and many of the people whose names are listed in the acknowledgments section. Of course, due to the impact of their assistance, we want to honor them. But, just as important are the lessons that some of their stories can offer people who are diagnosed with a terminal illness of their own.

DAN WIONS

extraordinary positive energy that simply attracts people to her. I, on the other hand, have for much of my life been rather strong willed and controlling, with a distinct sarcastic bent. Please don't let me mislead you, though. It's not that I see myself as some kind of over-bearing ogre (although some who know me well might argue in support of that view). It's just that I am not the angel my wife is.

My life goal and career endeavors have been focused on helping people achieve more satisfying and productive ways to approach their work and their lives. Along the way, it has been gratifying that people have credited me with having helped them achieve some significant and positive changes. I have always tried to be there for others and have made some contributions, of which I am quite proud. Some of my friends contend that this wealth of assistance that we are so fortunate to be receiving is merely payback: that I have somehow "earned" it. Yet, it continues to appear that the scales have tipped considerably in my favor. It feels as if I am getting back far more than I contributed.

My friend Nick, who often provides useful food for thought, has an interesting perspective on this. His take on what keeps this army of supporters parading through my life is that they get something very special out of it. Some may come for insight, some for inspiration, some for coaching, and some for the good feeling that comes from giving. Bob Fass, a long-time friend and another constant contributor to my well-being, often reminds me that I am doing a good deed—a *"mitzvah,"* as it is called in Jewish culture—by allowing someone to help. I get this. We are often moved to take action when witnessing others faced with difficult circumstances, and that is good for us. Being reminded of this makes it easier to be accepting when others are reaching out with offers of help. I also get why people would come for coaching, given that it has been a significant focus of my professional life for more than thirty years.

The one angle that I struggle with is the notion of being inspirational. I hear this often from people: that they are inspired by the strength and focus of the choice to live my life and pursue recovery, rather than curling up in depression and waiting to die. On a purely intellectual level, this is understandable. On an emotional level, however, it is sometimes a little embarrassing and difficult to accept. In my view, I am just a guy trying to survive an illness in the most deliberate way possible. Whatever the reasons why people keep coming, I am extremely grateful and live in constant wonder of the incredible depth, breadth, and consistency of the things they do for me, and my family.

• • •

I have said earlier that it was not surprising that my family stepped up with their love and support when they heard the diagnosis. It did not surprise me that they stepped up with financial support. It did not surprise me that they were willing to feed me when I could no longer handle utensils, or that they were willing to help answer the phone or make calls or help reposition me in the wheelchair. What did surprise me was the intensity and extensiveness of that support. Some made very generous and totally

> One of the most impressive things about Joe was how graciously and gracefully he managed an intolerable level of inconvenience and discomfort in the face of real suffering and extreme unpleasantness. I once saw him coach an individual who had suffered from depression and had attempted suicide. Joe, someone who fought for every inch of life, sat there and listened compassionately to someone who seemed willing to give it all up. He sat without anger or resentment, as an active listener and graceful coach. There was a "selflessness" in the way he approached difficulties that was and is a model for us all.
>
> **NICK KLEVANS**
> **HOSPICE VOLUNTEER,**
> **FRIEND**

unexpected monetary contributions to help us deal with the financial demands of my care. Others made extraordinary contributions of their time. Still others readily volunteered to help with personal hygiene issues that I never could have asked or expected of them.

My nephew, Josh Schreibman, is a good example. Over the years, we have become quite close, and he often seeks me out for guidance and advice. During the past few years, he has volunteered a considerable amount of his weekend time to provide breaks for my health aide and Diane. He has fed me, helped to dress me, assisted in answering e-mails, taken phone calls, clipped my fingernails, and more. The time that we spend together provides Josh with an opportunity to talk about his goals, aspirations, and obstacles— conversations that he finds helpful and I find rewarding. I am grateful that he lives close enough and is dedicated enough to provide so much valuable assistance—and that I can also help him in some way.

My brother-in-law, David Berg, and his wife, Jann, have also gone far beyond what I would have expected. David is my wife's younger brother who, with his unique wit, enormous heart, and strength of character has carved out a central role in our family. He and Diane have always been close. So, it was natural that he and Jann quickly showed up to help out. Their contributions, however, have been far beyond anything we could have expected—ranging from financial assistance to personal care. Despite living three hours away in Connecticut, they make it a point to visit several times a year to offer whatever help we need. During those visits, our home is filled with love and humor.

Many other family members have also stepped up to help out financially and physically. Some of them are limited by distance and some by their own health issues, but all have contributed with their love and intention. They include my mother-in-law, Bess Berg; my nephews, Eric and Michael Sherling, and their wives, Leslie and Dawn; my brother-in-law, Bruce Sherling, and his wife, Anna; my sister-in-law, Eileen Schreibman; and many other cousins, aunts, and uncles who are also listed in the acknowledgments of this book.

• • •

As with our family, friends have pitched in to help out in many different ways. With the progression of the disease, however, it has become more difficult for some of those friends to remain as engaged as they once were. This is understandable. When someone becomes physically limited, it alters the ways you can spend time together. Even something as simple as going to a movie or a restaurant becomes a formidable logistical challenge. People also have their own concerns to contend with and sometimes need to pull back in order to take care of themselves. Still others have so much difficulty watching a friend wrestle with a serious health issue that it is hard for them to be present in the situation.

And yet some friends, no matter what is going on in their lives, always seem to be there and are prepared to do whatever the moment requires. I remember a funny incident a few years ago while my pal Lenny and I were attending a Rutgers football game together. At the time, I was using a manual wheelchair to get around but still had fairly good use of my hands and arms. Nature called and I wheeled myself off to the men's room to take care of business. Upon my return, I shared with Lenny my dismay that it was getting increasingly difficult to manage the zipper on my pants in order to relieve myself. Without missing a beat, Lenny snapped back at the obvious implication, "That's where the friendship ends, buddy." Several years have now passed since that exchange, and Lenny has proven time and again that his commitment to our friendship is far deeper than his comical retort implied. (That is all I am saying.)

Walt and Zoe Fuller have been our good friends and neighbors for more than twenty years, and ALS has not changed that. If anything, it has drawn us closer. Whether it's helping to clean up a flooded basement, pulling weeds, spreading mulch, solving a computer problem, or painting a room, they are always there when needed, and often without being asked. Thanks to Walt and our adjacent neighbor, Raul Pedraja, and their trusty snow-blowers, we also never have to worry about being snowed in during the winter. In addition to doing chores for us, Walt and Zoe find plenty of time to join us for walks, include us at holiday barbecues, and come over with big bowls of popcorn to watch movies with us.

Diane's college roommates—Lisa Larson, Carol Dyer, and Phyllis Remoledor have been among our closest friends for almost forty years. While they live some distance away, they are frequently in touch, doing whatever they can to help out. Lisa and Carol travel from Massachusetts once or twice a year for a couple of days at a time to catch up on things, watch movies with us, provide foot massages, and pitch in with whatever is going on. Phyllis also visits from Florida whenever possible, and keeps in touch by e-mail.

> I remember late night summer swims with Joe. We discussed raising children, investment opportunities, creating high performing teams, playing tennis—which I would always let him win (that's my version of the story). We would also talk about childhood dreams. I found out that Joe loved to sing and had considered becoming a cantor. Who would have known?
>
> **JOEL LUBIN**
> CLOSE FRIEND

Joel and Jane Lubin have been part of our extended family since our children played together as toddlers over twenty years ago. Our visits have grown less frequent since their move to Maryland about ten years ago. Despite the distance, however, we are in constant contact and still manage to see each other several times a year. There is little I can think of that they would not or have not done for us.

One of the things I desperately miss is our summer vacations with them in Cape May, New Jersey. It was our tradition for nine years, until the energy drain and logistics of travelling with ALS made our rendezvous too difficult. By the summer of 2009, I had regained enough strength, energy and emotional balance to spark interest in trying to resurrect our tradition. After some intense investigation into managing equipment and access to buildings, however, it turned out that Joel and Jane's vacation house in Virginia was a longer ride but a much more manageable alternative. It was the longest trip we had made in almost four years, but worth every minute. In their typical loving and supportive way, Joel and Jane did everything imaginable to ensure my comfort, safety and access during the five days of our visit. Jane also made sure that I had all the organic produce needed to stay on track with my diet plan, and Joel handled personal care when my aide took his afternoon walks.

So, instead of watching the porpoises frolic in the surf while sunning ourselves on the beach at Cape May, we watched birds in their backyard while relaxing in their sunroom. We also took in the vistas and wildlife of Shenandoah National Park while driving along the Blue Ridge Parkway. We ate well, watched movies, talked, and most importantly, thoroughly enjoyed spending fun and uplifting times together.

My son, Dan, met his childhood best friend, David Stagg, in second grade, around the age of seven or eight. It did not take Dan long to fall in love with and adopt David's playful and fun-loving family as his own. At his urging, we invited the Staggs to go out to dinner with us. Before we knew it, we had practically been living in each other's homes for about the next eight years. David's sister, Jen, quickly evolved into Julie's "big sister," and their parents, John and Suzie, had an outrageously twisted and playful sense of humor. We skied together, barbequed together, spent holidays together, worked on projects together, attended each other's family events, and more.

After their move to Colorado, our visits were reduced to once or twice a year, usually in Colorado during the ski season. These trips ended when my legs gave out. Over the last few years, however, John and Sue have been making summertime visits with the express purpose of doing chores to help out. During their visits, Diane and Suzie would spend time together reorganizing the kitchen and all the closets in the house, and cleaning up the basement. John does carpentry work, electrical and mechanical repairs, chauffeuring, resolves computer problems, and even provides personal care when needed.

Our evenings are spent watching movies, chatting, and teasing each other. From the moment they walk in the door, it's as if we had seen them only yesterday. We relish every fun-filled and loving moment with them and are blessed to be able to count them among our closest friends.

In addition to the usual suspects, some other people have come forward unexpectedly to contribute extensive and amazing gifts. One such contributor is my good friend, Gil Gordon, who appeared out of nowhere after years of sparse contact and transformed himself from business acquaintance to something akin to a guardian angel. It all began with a phone call in September of 2003.

"Joe, this is Gil," said the voice on the other end of the phone. "I was reading an article about you in the Jewish State newspaper, and I was wondering if you'd be interested in getting together for lunch to catch up." The article that Gil was referring to had been initiated by my rabbi at the time, Shana Margolin. Her intention was to alert the local Jewish community about my situation in the context of my having been an active board member and volunteer in our congregation for many years. This phone call was evidence of the article's effectiveness.

Gil and I had worked in sister companies within the Johnson & Johnson organization. We had always been friendly and enjoyed each other's company, but had only seen each other maybe half a dozen times at professional meetings in the twenty-some years since those days. So it was a pleasant surprise to hear from him, and I readily took him up on his offer.

We had a lot of fun reminiscing about our common past, and how life had been treating us in the years since. It was so enjoyable, in fact, that we decided to schedule another lunch date.

During these conversations, it began to strike me how much we had

While finding and nurturing communities has been an essential part of building our support network, actually getting the message out to these communities has been just as important. When I think about the groups who have offered the most assistance (outside of close friends and family), four come to mind. They include our synagogue, Mom's students, Dad's colleagues, and our neighborhood. It wasn't always easy to ask for help directly.

However, often, just informing these groups of our situation was enough to ignite people into action. Gil is a perfect example of how effective that strategy was. The Jewish State Newspaper article was a great tool in this respect, as it got the message out to related communities with which my parents were less involved and less visible. In today's age of Facebook, Instagram, blogs, simple website templates, and Twitter, it's ridiculously easy to inform people of what's going on and stay in touch. The main concern is to determine how much privacy to relinquish. Get the word out, and people will flock to help.

DAN WIONS

in common that I had either overlooked or forgotten through the years. Gil and I were approximately the same age and each had two children (a boy and a girl) who were also about the same ages. We were both married to teachers, had both become consultants, and both enjoyed doing odd jobs with tools.

This last similarity took on a special significance during our second lunch meeting. I learned that Gil had taken his love for working with "man toys" a lot more seriously than I had. He was in the habit of contributing a considerable part of his typical week to working with Habitat for Humanity and was constantly on the prowl for projects that would provide him with an excuse to add to his arsenal of hand and power tools.

I expressed my looming concern about home maintenance chores that I would normally do myself. The instability in my legs was already making it a treacherous adventure to stand on a chair and change a light bulb. Handling tools like screwdrivers, hammers, and saws was on the verge of becoming too dangerous to consider. This was a growing reality that could contribute significantly to our financial burdens. Knowing this, Gil extended a very generous offer. He suggested that I keep a list of things that needed to be done around the house and call him when I had a few hours of work. He said he would be happy to volunteer his time and talents to help avert unnecessary expenses.

After our second lunch, Gil invited me to take a look at the trunk of his car. When he popped the lid, I found myself staring into what looked like a traveling hardware store. Not only were the tools bountiful in supply, but they were also impeccably organized and clean. The quantity and condition of the tools suggested that we shared a level of compulsiveness and similarity in work style that made me very comfortable with his playing handyman in my home. Over the past several years, Gil has done countless projects, saving me several thousands of dollars. He has become a regular fixture around my house and an indescribably good friend.

To leave you with the impression, however, that Gil's support has been limited to handyman status would truly be selling him short. He has provided just about every imaginable form of assistance. He has shopped, helped with internet searches, driven me to doctors' appointments, contributed financially, oriented and trained new health aides, and more. He has even performed as a health aide at times when there have been gaps in coverage. Gil has become my first line of defense whenever a home repair or health-aide crisis emerges. It is hard to describe the level of comfort derived from knowing that he is always there, ready and able to handle life's unexpected complications in a way that I would likely do it myself. The degree of stress that Gil's actions help to avoid is a direct and powerful contribution toward efforts to recover my physical wellness.

I often ponder what motivates Gil to keep on giving as much as he does. While I live in constant gratitude and awe of the number of people who have shown up unexpectedly to support me and my family through these difficult times, there are few who have matched the profound, wide-reaching perseverance of Gil's giving. As of this writing, he has been a relentless contributor toward my efforts to regain my health for almost seven years. About every six months, I am compelled to ask him if he ever regrets having gotten so involved, and what motivates him to continue. His answer is always the same. He has no regrets, and he is motivated by the awareness that a simple twist of fate could have easily reversed our roles.

Natalie London is another one of the delightful surprises in my army of supporters. At the onset of the illness, we had known each other for nearly twenty years as members of the same congregation. We had attended services and synagogue functions together many times over the years but had had little contact or association outside our temple. I knew her as a very pleasant, long-standing, and very involved member of the congregation but knew very little about her personally.

As my finger and hand functions began to deteriorate, there was an increasing need for help with filing, organizing, and computer matters. Natalie was one of the first to offer this kind of help. Her background as manager of a systems group, combined with a work style and attention to detail similar to my own, made her a perfect fit for this kind of help. She has become the main person I rely on to keep financial records in order, and to keep supplies ordered on time and organized. In addition, she has become one of my key go-to people when I need a ride or something picked up from the store. I often see her on a weekly basis or even multiple times a week, as she visits to drop off groceries or office supplies, helps out with paper or computer work, or plays chauffeur. Natalie has been providing this kind of support for about six years. While many have provided some of the same kind of help, few have been as consistent and enduring.

Perhaps the greatest blessing of Natalie's increased presence in my life has been the gift of her friendship. As we have gotten to know one another, we have discovered many shared interests, the most noteworthy of which are our mutual love of music and an undying dedication to our shared Jewish community. We have had many conversations about our children's musical adventures, and she has attended more than one performance at the high school where my wife teaches choral music. We also spend many hours discussing the activities, opportunities, and issues faced by our synagogue: everything from changes in leadership to the ebb and flow of membership to upcoming events. In the process, I have gotten to know her easy-going nature, her warmth, her caring, and her generosity. She has truly been an unexpected gift on the path down which ALS has taken me.

So many people contribute their time and resources to my care that they could be the subject of a separate book. Some friends visit regularly on weekends to provide time for my aide to get a break and for Diane to take care of things like laundry, shopping, and bills: people like Lee and Hope Schraeter; Li and Hong Jin and their son Nick; Hongbo Qi; Ling and Jake Song and their son, Kevin. Other friends, like Mike Divito and Tim Kowalski, have done everything from night duty when Diane is away to filling in as a health aide.

Some of these people are long-time friends. Others came to know me in the

> On occasion, we have the privilege of being touched by someone who not only inspires us, but challenges us to reflect on our own lives. This challenge is a gift, an opportunity to journey deep within ourselves and emerge with a clearer purpose and greater sense of who we are and how we fit in our local and global community. Joe is that rare person, the one who makes us all aspire to be the best we can be; I truly feel blessed and honored to call him my friend.
>
> **TIM KOWALSKI**
> LONGTIME FRIEND

battle with ALS. Some are students of Diane's and their parents. All are an inspiration, and I live in constant gratitude. I have devoted an Appendix to building a supportive community. I cannot emphasize enough how essential this has been for me.

CHAPTER FOURTEEN

The Blessing of Family

Not too long ago, I received an email requesting that I sign a petition to help a family in need of a new home to draw the attention of the *Extreme Makeover* TV show. A mother of two children was living with ALS in a small trailer. The husband had to quit his job to tend to his wife full time, since they could not afford health aides. How this family survived each day under such circumstances was beyond me. I have heard too many stories of families being torn apart by the pressures of dealing with a serious illness. I immediately signed the petition and sent it on to others, feeling heartbroken for this family and all the more blessed by my own circumstances. It is hard to imagine how we could survive as a family without a great deal of support.

My wife and children are recipients of support as much as I am. While others come, help out and leave, Diane, Dan and Julie live with the impact of my illness every day. We are fortunate to be able to afford health aides who take care of the bulk of my personal care. They cannot be available 24 hours a day, however; they do need breaks. Without assistance, the burden would fall on Diane and the kids to feed me, toilet me, answer phones, type, and handle a myriad of other details involved with my physical functioning. A day does not begin without my thanking God for my wife's and children's love and dedication.

Diane is a gifted choral music teacher who puts in enormously long hours between the regular school day, conferences, providing extra help to students, rehearsals, performances, and trips to competitions and music festivals to ensure success and profound personal growth experiences for her students. When she comes home from her twelve-to-fifteen-hour workdays, she can look forward to paying bills, doing laundry, shopping for groceries, writing college recommendations for her students, grading papers, and reviewing music for future rehearsals and performances. In between, she tries to squeeze in time for exercise at the gym or a power walk. Occasionally, we get to sit down and watch a movie together. At night, the five or six hours she has to sleep are often interrupted several times to help me urinate, make an adjustment on my breathing apparatus, scratch an itch, or help relieve a pain. Weekends are often consumed in large part by the household chores she can't get to during the week. In spite of all this, she has remained a loyal, dedicated, and loving partner who takes pleasure in simple things like watching a movie with me or soaking up some sunshine during the warmer months while holding a book for me to read. She has always been, and continues to be, one of the greatest blessings of my life.

While son and daughter do a great deal to contribute to my care, their efforts are limited by another challenge that we have faced as a family for more than twenty years. Both of them were diagnosed during childhood with Tourette's Syndrome, which I have also struggled with since my youth. Tourette's is a neurological disorder characterized by vocal and motor tics accompanied by obsessive-compulsive disorder. By early adolescence, both Dan and Julie had developed the rare symptom of sound sensitivity. When they would hear certain sounds, like the sharp pronunciation of the letter "s," for example, it produces a response in them of severe physical and emotional pain. While they do not react to everyone's sounds, they are particularly sensitive to mine and, to a slightly lesser degree, their mother's. As you can imagine, this can make it quite difficult for them to spend extended periods of time with me, especially if they are under stress. Given this situation, my children also benefit tremendously from the support we get from friends and family. And despite this obstacle, they both make amazing contributions to my care.

A few years ago, for example, when Dan travelled with me to Germany to see Dr. Kessler, I did what I could to avoid sounds that were difficult for him to handle. However, we were together for so much time that the inevitable would occur. When it did, Dan did whatever was necessary to manage his reactions and ensure that my well-being was never compromised. The dedication, love, and care that I received from him during that trip were nothing short of overwhelming.

Julie also has put in considerable time assisting in my care. She has cooked for and fed me, answered phones, and served as my arms and legs in innumerable ways. Despite her slender build, she possesses great strength, and has even helped to transfer me to and from my wheelchair and bed.

It is not an easy thing for a child to watch a disease reduce a parent to almost half his physical size. I have had many conversations with both Dan and Julie in which we have helped each other cope with the powerful impact that ALS and Tourette's have had on our lives and our relationships. They have helped me every bit as much as I have helped them in extracting growth from an enormous challenge. I am a very proud father.

. . .

I believe that 2006 was the first year in which I could no longer use the stair glide to ascend the six steps from our den to the kitchen/dining room level of our home. Generally, this is not a significant issue, since the aides prepare my meals and bring them to me. At special family gatherings like Thanksgiving, however, being absent from the dining area takes on more psychological and emotional significance. Sitting immobile in the midst of the hustle and bustle of twenty family members running around the house, catching up on each other's lives, it's easy to experience moments of feeling left out or overlooked. I have to remind myself that the day isn't just about me. I have to take responsibility for engaging others in conversation, and feeling appreciated when others reach out to me—which they frequently do. But when the tribe migrates upstairs to the dining room, and I am unable to join them on such an important family day, well...

Before we installed the stair glider, my son provided the remedy to this problem. He simply picked me up out of the wheelchair and carried me up the steps to the dining room, where he gently deposited me in another wheelchair. The rock-hard muscles of his sculpted arms cradled me with the security of a pair of padded iron bars. His powerful legs propelled us up the stairs as easily as if he were carrying a bag of groceries.

The first time he did this, I couldn't help but reflect in awe on the miracle of life. It seemed like only yesterday that Diane had blessed me with a beautiful red-haired, blue-eyed wonder that we chose to name Daniel. I remember hovering over the bed in the recovery room, mesmerized by the miracle that Diane and I had created, and overwhelmed and dazed by the flood of love, pride, gratitude, and awe that was rushing through me. My mind raced forward through a myriad of treasured moments during his infant and toddler years when I would lift him over my head in play, and revel in his squeals of delight. It was almost unimaginable that this tiny little creature whom I had once carried in the palm of one hand was the same person who was now so easily and lovingly carrying me up the stairs.

Tuesdays with Morrie, Mitch Albom's account of his beloved professor's demise from ALS, is filled with many touching and insightful moments. One that I found particularly moving and relevant was when Morrie talked about the importance of a family's love. "This is part of what a family is about, not just love. It's knowing that your family will be there watching out for you. Nothing else will give you that. Not money. Not fame. Not work."

I am reminded of the holiday times when Diane, Julie, or Dan would either orchestrate or engage in the act of carrying me upstairs to the dining room to ensure my inclusion. It reminds me of the times when one or all of them would come flying down the stairs to assist me if an aide was not responding quickly enough to my coughing or choking. It brings to mind how they rarely enter or leave the house without making sure to plant a kiss on my forehead as they come and go. I feel blessed by their love, and rest with the knowledge that they are always looking out for me.

> Back In 2009, Joe agreed to speak to my students at Hillsborough High School about his experience with ALS. They had read *Tuesdays with Morrie*, and Joe trekked out to spend an entire afternoon at the school, answering the students' questions and sharing his wisdom. Typical Joe: going out of his way to help others.
>
> **RICHIE BENCIVENGA**
> CLOSE FRIEND OF JULIE

CHAPTER FIFTEEN

The Gift of Community

A sense of community is something that has been important to me for most of my adult life. I have had the good fortune to have experienced the rewards of community involvement in a wide variety of forms, including family, shared friendships, neighborhood, work relationships, township of residence, religious congregation, and more. It is my strong belief that we accomplish little in life alone and that by honoring our connections to others we enrich our own lives as well as those to whom we offer help and support. In each of the communities in which I participate, I have always found it to be extremely rewarding to contribute my time, talents, and energies in the service of others. ALS has provided me with an opportunity to experience the rewards of community from a different and very powerful perspective. One community in particular supported me and my family through this odyssey.

> There is something about our big Township that really feels like a small town. It keeps us in touch over the long haul—a community of caring neighbors and friends. Few people I know could have endured the challenges that have faced you. I believe that this town and the people who have come to know you and pull for you have added to the strength, determination and courage you have shown. Our roots are firmly set in a wonderful community to raise a family, to raise the spirit, and to raise the devil as needed. Joe, you are proof that an optimistic heart and soul will beat the odds. Live strong.
>
> **BILL FOELSCH**
> LONGTIME FRIEND

My religious community, Congregation Kehilat Shalom (CKS), formerly known as the Jewish Community Center of Belled Mead, stepped up in some startling ways. The board established a fund to provide members facing financial issues due to loss of employment or extreme illness with additional monetary resources. I was lucky to have purchased disability insurance when I'd started my business a decade before I got sick, but, as the next few years unfolded, there were mountains of unanticipated costs. The support of CKS was instrumental in helping to pay for home modifications, adaptive equipment, and therapies that I might otherwise have had to forego.

In addition to financial assistance, members organized to provide meals and groceries on an ongoing basis. They also contributed their time to help with record keeping, yard work, transportation, and household chores.

• • •

I don't consider myself a devoutly religious man, but I do identify quite strongly with my Jewish heritage and sense of community. CKS has had a lot to do with that. As an active congregant for twenty-plus years, a former board member, and a past president, I have witnessed firsthand the miracles that emerge when a community of people truly supports one another. My personal experience has been that the more I have

> "If I closed my eyes and didn't see the wheelchair or Bi-PAP, half the time I'd think I was having a pastoral counseling session with Joe, and not the other way around. He has been a wise and caring friend and I am grateful to know him."
>
> **RABBI SUSAN FALK**
> LONGTIME FRIEND

given to this community, the more I seem to get back. Following my diagnosis, I was surprised at how awkward I felt, at first, in the role of receiver. It has taken a while to feel that it is okay for me to be the focus of their gifts. To be honest, I am still learning to be totally accepting. Over time, I have come to realize that accepting such gifts completes an exchange in which both parties benefit. I receive something that makes my physical and emotional issues more manageable, and the giver gets to feel the blessing of having made a positive difference in another person's life.

During the process of this evolution in my thinking, I have been in awe of the abundant blessings that result when such exchanges are allowed to flourish. I have humbly watched people learn and grow through their exposure to my situation, and I have been overwhelmed with the outpouring of love and support that my family and I have received from friends, relatives, and even strangers.

One of the most impressive things about the efforts of my fellow congregants is their sustained committment. It is natural and understandable that, when there is an extended period of need, people's busy lives make it hard to provide ongoing support over the long haul. Many of the people who initially signed up to provide meals, for example, have fallen off the list of active participants, yet others have stepped in to take their places. Still others have continued to participate in this way for several years: my long-time friends, Bob and Peggy Fass, Marc and Harlene Rosenberg, Sheryl and Richard Rosenberg, Tobie and Stan Parnett, and Debbie Lampf are among those who have endured while others have come and gone.

Sheryl has also been extremely helpful in coordinating a lot of the work contributed by other members of our community. Month after month, she sends out the e-mails to find out who is available to bring food or groceries. Once the responses are in, Sheryl and I review the possibilities and put together a schedule which she then e-mails back to those who have offered their time. She has been doing this like clockwork for more than three years, while coordinating other efforts on my behalf as well.

My friend, Bob, in addition to helping out with food and groceries, makes frequent visits to check in with me, often bringing some classic comedy movie with him to make sure I get my quota of humor therapy. Marc and Natalie are always on call to provide transportation or make runs to the grocery store. Meryl Orlando and Randi Katzman take care of any tailoring needs as well as contributing to meal and grocery supplies. Matt Rosenthal, our current president, and our rabbi, Susan Falk, make regular visits to check on my progress, keep me apprised of temple issues and developments, and to exchange ideas. The list goes on and on....

• • •

Another group that has provided valuable support in my adventures with ALS is the medical community with which I am affiliated. While most of my efforts in dealing with this illness have been in the realm of alternative medicine, these groups have played significant roles in helping me to understand ALS and to maintain my functionality and wellness.

Each progression of the illness has come with the loss of some physical ability. The first thing to go was my ability to run. Then came the day when I could no longer walk without the aid of some orthopedic device. My legs becoming too weak to operate the pedals of my car was a huge blow, and when my hands could no longer hold a pen or a fork, or operate a keyboard, that was also nearly devastating. Over the years, I lost all ability to stand or walk, and with each physical loss, another element of my independence evaporated. I became increasingly reliant on others to accomplish basic tasks of daily living.

The Philadelphia Chapter of the ALS Association (ALSA) and the neurology clinic of Dr. Leo McCluskey at the University of Pennsylvania Hospital have played huge roles in helping me through some of these transitions. They have provided a constant source of devices and recommendations to help with the evolving physical constraints. This has even included braces to help keep my fingers straight, to facilitate pulling on my socks, buttoning my shirts, and eating. The Philadelphia ALSA also guided me to people who could advise me on home alterations that could increase my accessibility. When getting in and out of bed became difficult, they got me a hospital bed. They provided counseling, when needed, to help me and my family get through the rough spots. And when my breathing got below 30 percent of vital capacity, they guided me to hospice and introduced me to the concept in a way that mitigated the intimidating implications of becoming a hospice patient.

For several years, the Philadelphia ALSA provided significant financial assistance in the area of home health care. As my physical deterioration outpaced my family's ability to provide for my daily care, we became increasingly reliant on the services of home health aides to fill in the gaps. It didn't take much before we were spending several hundreds of dollars per week for this kind of support—our single most consistent financial challenge. Without the partial relief we got from

ALSA's home health aide program, it would have been nearly impossible to have afforded the necessary help. While they continue to support me in other ways, recent budgetary cutbacks have forced Philadelphia ALSA to discontinue subsidization of home health care. Fortunately, we have found other more affordable ways to secure the help I desperately need.

· · ·

Once I became a hospice patient, some of the services provided through ALSA and the neurology clinic in Philadelphia were taken over by the hospice organization. Among them were things like payments for durable medical equipment, and the services of a nurse, social worker, and a respiratory therapist—a delightful young woman by the name of Julie Seifert, who shows up once a month with her bright demeanor to check my breathing equipment and my breathing capacity. Julie has been extremely helpful in evolving my understanding of my breathing-capacity measures, the equipment that I use to support it, and in keeping me positively focused on the implications of the numbers we get each month.

My hospice nurse, Maureen Woods, has become a true partner in helping me to manage the ancillary physical issues of ALS—things like aches and pains, rashes, sleeplessness, and, let's just say, temporary dysfunctions of my metabolism. She has also become a key asset in helping me to assess physical and emotional changes resulting from alternative medical strategies that I have employed. As days go by, it can be difficult to keep track of the subtle changes in your body's functioning and your own attitude and outlook when dealing with a chronic illness. Maureen's openness to my experiments with alternative approaches and her attentiveness to these changes have

> Joe has the best interest of his loved ones (and that's just about everyone) at the forefront of his struggles and allows their joys and experiences to enrich his life.
>
> And ALS? That's a disease that Joe has. It isn't who he is.
>
> **MAUREEN WOODS**
> **HOSPICE NURSE**

provided an invaluable perspective, as well as stability in tracking the results of my efforts.

Another enlistee in the hospice army of supporters is my social worker, Liz Cohen. About once a month, Liz shows up at my door to check in and see how things are going. She has a gentle and caring demeanor that provides an easy context in which to explore anything that may be troubling me. Whenever something comes up that threatens my resolve to recover, I look forward to a visit from Liz as an opportunity to break through the funk and get back on track.

One of the most amazing parts of the hospice experience is the array of volunteer contributors. These people donate their time out of the pure goodness of their hearts to make life easier for dying (or in my case, stubbornly NOT dying) patients. Some are retired. Others volunteer their time in addition to working full-time jobs. All are remarkable people. Through the hospice volunteer program, Nick has contributed to my well-being through his integrative therapy work and his stimulation of my spiritual development. Roger Holdredge and JoAnn Ferraro have enabled me to read books through their weekly visits to turn pages for me. Last but not least, Joan Montanari's dedicated weekly visits to type for me are what have made this book a reality. Perhaps the most essential support that hospice has provided me on a daily basis is the twenty hours a week of care from a home health aide. As my physical capabilities have declined, this service has become more and more valuable and important to my daily functioning. At the time of this writing, I am currently dependent on live-in care. The four hours of care each weekday provided by hospice ensures critical break time for my private-pay live-in aide. Tending to a person whose level of paralysis leaves him dependent on another for almost all tasks of daily living can be physically and emotionally draining. The amount of lifting, fetching, preparing, organizing, cleaning, and simply acting as a second pair of hands can keep a health aide busy for hours on end. Without sufficient time to take care of his or her own needs, a live-in aide can get worn down in a hurry, so the break time provided by a hospice aide has been essential.

· · ·

In addition to my congregation, medical community, extended family, and colleagues, I must acknowledge the educational community that revolves around my wife's work as a high school choral teacher. This wonderful group of students and parents provides everything from weekend health-aide relief, financial contributions, and food preparation, to yard work, organizing fundraisers, and producing benefit concerts. The intense demands of caring for someone with a serious illness can be a source of burnout for even the most dedicated and well-intentioned helpers. We are truly blessed to have the extensive and committed support of these communities working on our behalf to help avoid this danger.

CHAPTER SIXTEEN

March of the Health Aides

While I remained fairly self-sufficient with ALS for quite some time, I found myself becoming more and more dependent on others as my manual dexterity diminished. With the help of friends, I was able to keep up with things like filing and paperwork, but other tasks of daily living were becoming much too difficult, and I could only rely on friends to do so much. Consequently, I became increasingly dependent on paid home health care.

By the fall of 2004, I was employing health aides for three to four hours each morning to get me ready for the day. Within a year, as my ability to actively participate diminished, it would take an aide six hours to complete the same tasks, and by that time I required additional assistance into the afternoon. In June 2005, with my admission into hospice, came the relief of an additional twenty hours a week of insurance-covered home health care. By the end of 2005, I was requiring assistance morning, noon, and night. By the spring of 2006 it became necessary to hire a live-in to ensure 24/7 coverage.

While it was a great relief to have regular and reliable help, the increasing reliance on home health aides came with some emotionally and psychologically challenging issues. Among these issues was the increasing financial burden. Although assistance from the Philadelphia ALSA helped to mitigate this burden, securing this assistance required the use of the more expensive state-approved agencies. It took me a long time to stop beating myself up for neglecting the decision to purchase long-term-care insurance. Nevertheless, we adjusted and managed to cover the costs for the help we needed.

Even more difficult than the monetary costs, however, were the personal adjustments. Typically, when you hire someone for a job, you conduct interviews, look for a good fit, and make a choice among various options. Most health aide agencies, however, operate differently. You provide them with your criteria, then they do a search and assign a health aide. So when that stranger shows up at your door, you only have a short window of time between "Hi, how are you?" and "Would you mind bringing me that bottle, and putting my member in it, so I can take a pee?" It takes some work, just on a personal level, to get through the self-esteem and pride issues involved in such a situation. On the one hand, you might feel a deep sense of relief and gratitude that you have someone who is willing to help. At the same time, however, you can be overcome with feelings of extreme exposure and vulnerability. This is not an easy balancing act.

Adding to the difficulty is the fact that most aides come from different cultural and language backgrounds. These differences can create a rather awkward situation when you are having trouble with your breathing equipment and your aide can't understand what you need him to do. Often, an aide may have a widely different set of interests, communication habits, and understanding of priorities. Little things, like how you want your clothing organized to save time telling new caregivers where to find things, or picking a TV program that works for both of you, can become unneeded sources of tension. Add to this the occasional dilemma of clashes in personality or values, and you have the potential for a level of stress that isn't exactly conducive to healing. When you spend the better part of every day with a person upon whom you are dependent for all of your activities of daily living, you want the relationship to be easy and enjoyable. You also have to consider the comfort level of your family, whose privacy is also being invaded by each new stranger to your domain.

Of course, if it's not working out you can always request that the agency send you a different aide, but such an exchange comes with several issues. First, you are still dependent on the one you've got until a replacement arrives, and a sour attitude can affect care. Second, the training of a new aide in your routine and physical handling takes considerable time and effort, and care often suffers during the learning process. Third and worst of all, you often don't know for several weeks if the new aide will be any better than the one he or she replaced. If the care is no better, you can find yourself starting all over again!

It took me a couple of years of spiritual growth, and physical healing to break through some of the myths I had locked myself into that made this situation even more difficult. I had to sort out my complex feelings around being so vulnerable and dependent. I had to let go of my belief that there was no perfect aide and that I would always have to settle. And I had to let go of my fear and prejudice that dealing with less expensive, non-state-certified agencies put me and my family at risk of being exposed to less-skilled and less-trustworthy aides.

While evolving my way through these and other limiting beliefs, I witnessed the turnover of an incredible parade of caregivers marching through my home. Although a few were either so personally objectionable or incompetent that we had to remove them quickly, most of them left for a myriad of their own reasons. The rigors of the job of caring for someone who is ninety percent paralyzed are but one of a number of contributing factors. I have lost aides due to injuries, to go back to school, to seek other types of employment, to address family issues, and more.

In the four years that I have been dependent on home care, I have worked with more than twenty health aides. A few of them stand out and have genuinely contributed to the advancement of my health. My very first hospice aide, a registered nurse from Colombia, probably spoiled me for many that followed her. I am guessing that it was a combination of Luz's unpolished English skills and the need to support two young daughters as a single mom that she never pursued recertification as a nurse in the U.S. It was clearly to my advantage, however, to have someone with the depth and breadth of her skill base as my health aide.

In addition to her skills, Luz brought a personality that was worthy of her name, which in Spanish means "light." For six months, she brought light into my life every day. Always upbeat, she had a great sense of humor, and was very easy to deal with whenever confusion or misunderstanding came into play. When time permitted, we would watch the travel channel together while conversing half in Spanish and half in English. Being in the presence of her spirit was an elevating and healing experience. Sadly, an injury to her wrist, sustained while caring for another patient, brought our relationship to a premature end. Several aides and several months later, Lloyd entered my life for four years—longer than any other aide has been with me. As it was with Luz, there was never a task too large, too small or too unpleasant to discourage him from providing me with the best possible care.

There are many aides who, as immigrants to this country, take on this work because it is one of the best-paying jobs they can find. Despite this, some do the work quite well. But then there are those who do this kind of work because it is their calling to care for people who cannot care for themselves. The level of compassion and sensitivity to the needs of the patient demonstrated by such people sets them apart.

Lloyd was a soft-spoken, easy-going, and lovable soul who cared deeply about people. I got the greatest kick out of watching movies with him in which someone was being denied something that he deserved. Lloyd's intolerance of injustice drew him into such intense sympathy with the character that I would constantly find myself reminding him, "Lloyd, it's just a movie!"

Lloyd was a wonderful companion and a staunch supporter of my quest for recovery. We would talk about everything from our children's adventures to alternative therapies to politics. He was always willing to support me, no matter how far "out of the box" my alternative methods took me. He was also one of my greatest cheerleaders, always reminding me of his conviction that I would one day rise up out of this wheelchair and walk again.

Another of my extraordinary caregivers was a Kenyan man by the name of Jeremiah. During the year of my greatest decline, he would show up shortly after Diane left for work to help me with my morning ablutions, which doubled from a three to a six-hour process.

Each day with Jeremiah began with a loud and cheery "How are you today, young man?" His greeting always tickled me, both for the positive charge that it put in the air, and because we were about the same age. We had great chemistry fueled by a number of shared values and interests. Even politics was a safe topic of discussion for us.

Jeremiah was with me the day I lost the use of my right leg. It was a painfully memorable experience, both physically and emotionally. Jeremiah's handling of the situation revealed a great deal about the depth of his character and the kind of person he was.

It was a beautiful sun-bathed morning in the early fall of 2005. Multi-colored, dew-drenched leaves glistened in the morning light, and an out-of-season hummingbird buzzed around the feeder. The lightness of mood generated by the sunbeams pouring in through my bedroom window stood in sharp contrast to the intensity of trauma I was about to experience. Jeremiah and I had finished my range-of-motion exercises and had begun working our way through the bathroom routines.

I was in the process of transferring myself from my wheelchair to the shower seat, a process which I had been doing successfully for several months. It involved hoisting myself out of the chair on my arms, balancing myself mostly on my stronger left leg while reaching for grab bars on either side of me, turning myself toward the shower seat, and then lowering myself onto it with one hand on the seat and the other on the grab bar. As I was turning myself toward the shower seat, my right leg gave out without warning. In a split second, I was lying crumpled on the shower floor, with my right foot forced up against the wall and my knee in a hyper-flexed position. The sound of tearing ligaments as I fell was as scary as the pain was excruciating. As the fog of impending unconsciousness clouded my senses, all that filled my awareness was the fear of physical damage, the throbbing pain in my knee, the rush of emotion, and Jeremiah leaping into action.

In as short an instant as it had taken me to fall, Jeremiah scooped me up in his arms like a baby and carried me to my bed. He quickly covered me to keep me warm and did whatever was necessary to get me comfortable and help me recover from the immediate trauma. I vaguely recall my legs being raised and an ice pack somehow finding its way onto my knee. As my mind and body calmed and my awareness grew clearer, I began to notice that Jeremiah, though doing everything right, was extremely upset. He kept apologizing profusely for allowing me to fall, as if there were some way he could have actually prevented it. Even though he had been standing right next to me, the fall was so sudden that no human being could have reacted in time to prevent it. What I remember more than fear or the pain, is the depth and breadth of Jeremiah's compassion and care in getting me through the traumatic experience.

Among my aides, Jesse Moko, who was with me for eight months, also set a standard that few others have been able to match. He came with an extraordinary set of skills, far beyond the credentials of most health aides. Jesse was also from Kenya, where he worked for twenty years as a registered nurse. His cleanliness, organizational skills, and knowledge of how to care for the human body created a sense of security and reliability that far exceeded what I had experienced with most others. In addition, a strong appreciation for family, extremely professional manner, and a positive and pleasant demeanor made him a very comfortable member of our household.

I knew, almost from the day he arrived, that his talent would only be on loan to me for a limited period of time. Jesse was one of the most focused people I have ever met. During the time he was with me, I watched him meticulously organize and implement a clear and deliberate plan for his career and his family's needs. He spent his time off during his first five months with me studying for the nursing boards, which he easily passed. After that, it was just a matter of time until he found the nursing job he sought in San Diego. It was a difficult parting for both of us on the day he left.

Apart from Luz, Lloyd, Jeremiah, and Jesse, I experienced a wide range of skills and qualities in my caregivers. Each relationship had its strengths and weaknesses. Some of the weaknesses were quite startling, and disappointing. I had caregivers whose attention would remain glued to the TV while I was choking on a piece of food from my dinner. Some would leave me at risk for several minutes when angered over a misunderstanding. Others would press me for instructions on how to help during times when I was short of air, not having the sense to put my Bi-PAP back in place to enable me to speak. Through their strengths and weaknesses, I learned something from every one of them. In some cases, the learning was joyful. In others, it was painful. But in all cases, it was valuable. With each new relationship, I grew increasingly clear about the skills and attributes I required in an aide to ensure appropriate care.

Perhaps the most important lesson I learned is that I don't have to settle. Despite the intense investment of time and energy to train a health aide, it's better to start over sooner rather than later. I learned how valuable a good caregiver is to my well-being, and that the definition of "good" includes personality fit as well as skill sets. With the right health aide, vulnerability and stress are reduced to a minimum, allowing me to focus my energies on healing rather than surviving. The "right fit" for me is that someone who is organized and neat, with a good sense of humor, a willingness to communicate, and who is secure enough to resolve misunderstandings without upset.

In February 2009, as a result of an apparent crisis that turned out to be a blessing in disguise, I found my "perfect aide." It began with the call from the ALS Association that they were discontinuing my home health care. This forced me to start looking at the less expensive, non-state-certified agencies. As a result of this search, Gintaras (Jimmy) Franka walked into my life. Despite lacking the official credentials, Jimmy arrived with all the skills, willingness, and personality to support me in maintaining a joyful outlook on life and to ensure my safety and well-being.

I feel quite fortunate to have had the opportunity, prior to my illness, to develop the verbal and teaching skills that enabled me to cope with and learn from a wide variety of caregiver experiences with considerably less stress than would otherwise have been possible. I also feel blessed to have had such a diverse group of people show up willingly at my door to perform the very personal work of being my home health aide. Through my experiences with them I have gained patience, tolerance, adaptability, humility, and more. I have included all of my advice for seeking home care into an Appendix.

CHAPTER SEVENTEEN:
Blessings in Disguise
Growing Through Challenge

Blessings don't always look or feel like blessings. Sometimes the insight derived from a bad situation, or the change that emerges from it, turns out to be a valuable gift. When someone forces you to look at a behavior or thought pattern that does not serve you well—or may even be causing you damage—the experience can be quite uncomfortable. If, however, you can muster the courage to acknowledge, own, and change your dysfunctional pattern, this temporary discomfort transforms into a positive insight. Having had several of these experiences in recent years, I have become more attuned to looking for and appreciating the blessings in disguise.

One of the first examples is the experience I had with my first live-in health aide. Although Ethan (not his real name) possessed a number of very positive attributes, it soon became apparent that he had some personal characteristics that made me increasingly uncomfortable, and which impinged on the quality of my care. He had very strong opinions, and a degree of self-absorption that demonstrated little regard for the emotional impact of his behaviors on others. He also had a tendency to move quickly and unnecessarily from discussion to argument when offered an alternative perspective.

My increasing discomfort with these behavior patterns brought into sharp focus my biggest problem in dealing with this first stranger in our midst: I was totally dependent upon him for all my basic activities of daily living, and at the mercy of this man, who was becoming increasingly emotionally abusive. I felt helpless and trapped, believing that if I called the agency it might not be possible to find an immediate replacement. These feelings were compounded by two other complicating factors—one being the additional stress it would create for Diane to take off from work to care for me until a replacement was found, and the other was the fear of further inciting Ethan's dysfunctional behavior, making his remaining time with me even more difficult. In addition I could not make a phone call without his assistance.

This aide was with us for just under three months, but it seemed much longer. Our relationship came to an end on a day in late June that, by no coincidence, happened to be Diane's last day of work for the school year. Ethan had launched into a prolonged tirade over a question I had asked him while he was showering me that morning.

He had already informed me of his plans to move on to a different type of work and had promised me considerable notice for finding a replacement. While I was appreciative of this, I was also concerned that a replacement, once found, might not be able to wait until Ethan was ready to leave. I shared this concern with him and asked if we could explore other options that would protect him financially if a replacement was ready to start before his planned departure.

He interpreted my inquiry as an offensive attempt to violate our "agreement" about the terms of his departure and commenced to rail at me as if I had just threatened his mother's life. His tirade lasted well over an hour despite my efforts to clarify my intention and despite efforts to remind him that he was creating an intolerable level of stress for a neurologically impaired patient whose care was his responsibility. His rant evolved into anger over how unappreciative I was and threats over how difficult it was going to be to replicate the quality of his care.

Bolstered by the knowledge that Diane would be home for the summer within hours, eliminating the threat of being left without care, and having reached my breaking point, I screamed at him, with expletives included, exactly what I thought of the quality of his care. Ironically, it was my lashing back that took the wind out of his sails and calmed him down. He was so "hurt" by my comments that he decided he could no longer work with me and would have to leave immediately. I was both shocked and relieved by this sudden turn of events. We called the agency together and explained what happened.

Ethan left that afternoon, and a replacement was provided the very next day.

Given the intensity of this episode, it could probably be argued that Ethan's tirade was anything but a blessing, so let me explain why I see it as such. The gifts that Ethan left me were a heightened awareness of my fears about being vulnerable and an opportunity to reality-test and mitigate those fears. I also learned that, while I was physically limited, I was not helpless. There were subsequent aides who also did not work out well and needed to be replaced. Yet I never again feared the changing of the guard or being left without care in the process. I discovered that we had friends, family members, and multiple agencies that we could count on to step in and fill the breach, if necessary, when transitioning to a new aide. This experience made me more aware of the support and resources available, and how only fear could prevent me from exercising my power to deploy them.

Through the three-month stretch with this aide, I learned these very important lessons: I am not at anyone's mercy. I do not need to be driven by fear. I have many resources available to me and the power to use them.

So, rather than demonizing Ethan, I choose to remember him with gratitude for providing me with a powerful, if painful, learning opportunity that helped me develop a much calmer, more deliberate, and more effective manner of dealing with life's crises.

> Joe came to my professional rescue back in 2002 when he agreed to audit, diagnose, and treat the management team at my company. His counsel, interventions, training and development made a huge difference. We were able to turn around our communication process and head toward success. Without Joe, I would not have been able to stay in that role, or be at all effective. Joe's guidance empowered me to make a big impact and keep the company on track. I learned a tremendous amount about organizations, communication, and myself in the process. During that time, Joe also became a dear friend and trusted mentor. I know his words will continue to make a difference in people's lives the way they have in mine.
>
> **LISA KENT**
> LONGTIME FRIEND

• • •

Some blessings arrive only partially disguised. Tom was a good example of this, the Tom who came with his partner, Tamara, to guide me through the use of the lemonade diet, the Colema Board, essential oils, etc. Probably the most critical contribution Tom made to the healing process was in helping to develop my consciousness of the mind/body interaction.

In a very short period of time, he made me painfully aware of how my thinking processes were contributing to my demise. He was extremely effective at getting in my face about the use of words that revealed defeatist thinking and expectations of death. It was shocking to discover, for example, how often variations of the word "try" had crept in to my conversation. I was constantly "trying" different healing modalities, "trying" to understand instructions, "trying" to use more affirmative words when I spoke. Phrases I had been accustomed to using most of my life, like "that makes me crazy," or "I'm dying to see that happen," suddenly became reflections of my deepest intentions and expectations for the outcome of my illness. These phrases seemed innocent enough, and at times I thought Tom was making too much of it. But he was relentless in pointing out how words like "crazy" and "dying" connected to the status of my health and expectations for the future. He was equally relentless in pointing out how words like "trying" automatically implied the expectation of potential failure.

I had invited Tom to come into my life with new strategies for healing that I knew were intended to shake up my world, and he was doing his job very effectively. The problem was that I had quickly reached a point where I was afraid to open my mouth. I was beginning to feel as if I couldn't say anything right. For a man who had spent thirty years of his life earning his living on the strength of his communication skills, this was a severely confounding and debilitating predicament. I became increasingly agitated every time Tom called me on a word that reflected my dysfunctional thinking.

While he remained unwaveringly effective in pointing out my use of negative words, he was not providing much help in learning a new and healthier vocabulary. It felt as if he had ripped out my tongue and left me to figure out for myself how to achieve the impossible task of growing back a new and better one. I felt clueless, helpless, antagonized, and even "paralyzed" by his approach. It did not occur to me until several years later that the response to Tom's technique was so intense because it reflected my worst fears about the ultimate toll that ALS could take. One night, about half way through the two-week period that Tom and Tamara spent under my roof, I reached the breaking point. It started off with him "nailing" me one more time about "trying" something. I pushed back, insisting that, while I could accept his premise that the overuse of these words was counterproductive, and even harmful, it was difficult to believe that I needed to completely eliminate them from my vocabulary. I was convinced I could find some use of the word "try" that was not unhealthy to employ. Tom wouldn't give an inch. At this point, paralysis evoked rage. Protest quickly evolved into a tirade fueled by intolerable levels of frustration. Suddenly, I was screaming profanities at him. The rant lasted far longer than it was reasonable to expect any human being to tolerate. Tom would have been perfectly within his rights to scream back or to get up and leave. To his credit, he did neither. He sat there calmly—and probably a little in shock—and he listened.

I don't remember how we left things that evening, but by the next morning we were treating each other very differently. As a result of the blowup, we had reached a clearer understanding of the changes that were needed in our communication to take me to the next level of learning. Tom confronted me less frequently about the use of words. When he did, however, it was clearer that he was merely holding up a mirror. I realized he was not now, nor had he ever been, judging me for using negative terminology. He was simply creating awareness. My own judgments and fears had been fueling frustrations and anger. I don't know if it was part of Tom's plan all along to drive me to that point, or if there was something he needed to learn about how to give more constructive and developmental feedback. Perhaps it was a little of each. Regardless of how we got there, from that point on I was a changed man.

Thanks to Tom's tolerance and his willingness to adapt along with me, lessons emerged from this experience that launched me into a new and highly productive phase of healing. It finally became clear that much of my frustration was driven by fear of the difficulty in transforming a core part of my identity and self-worth. My communication skills had been fundamental to my career success. To discover that aspects of these skills were actually contributing to my potential death was almost too difficult to face. It was much easier to focus on Tom's limitations in providing feedback. It was much easier to argue against stopping the use of certain words. It was much easier to accuse Tom of being insensitive and too extreme.

With this revelation came others, not the least of which was a new awareness of the degree to which my control issues had grown. It was certainly not through this process that I discovered I was a control freak; friends and family had devoted relentless effort for many years to make me aware of this characteristic. What I came to realize in working with Tom was how my feelings of being helpless to avert this race toward impending doom were causing me to over-control everything else in life. And with this awareness came freedom.

Suddenly, it became alright to throw out old work files without going through each page—it no longer felt as if I were throwing away my life; I was merely turning a page to a new chapter. No longer did I concern myself about whether we were down to our last banana. Someone else could worry about the shopping, and there would be something else to eat if there were no bananas.

Instead of worrying, controlling, and judging, I began focusing on building a new, healthy vocabulary, thinking about living, and creating a future, rather than anticipating and planning for my demise. Days now began with the recitation of a gratitude list and affirmations about the abundance of positives in my life. Conversation was now characterized by affirming words like "living," "doing," and "becoming." There was now time in the day to read again, and to take mental trips to the gym, training my brain to signal my muscles to move again.

Tom showed up at a time when I was feeling desperate and out of options. He challenged me to walk down a path that was both scary and deeply desirable. That path led to highways of discovery in the pursuit of healing. I shall forever be indebted to him for the patience, strength, tolerance, and courage he displayed by standing in the face of my fire and allowing me to grow from it.

THE DEFINING MOMENT

Evolution can take tens of thousands of years to occur. I don't think any of us will ever forget the day it happened in the span of an hour for my dad. After a week of figurative head butting, Tom took a new approach, in the form of a visualization exercise. The following is paraphrased:

Tom: Joe, were your parents at all abusive when you were a child?

Dad: Well, my mom certainly had her limitations, but she did the best she could. I don't think she was particularly abusive, no.

Tom: Can you think of a time, a specific example, when you were really angry with your mom?

Dad: Sure. I couldn't have been more than 9 years old. Some of my neighborhood friends invited me to go play by the creek one late summer afternoon. I went in to ask my Mom if I could go. She said sternly that I couldn't because it was getting late, and she didn't want me getting dirty before dinner. I was really upset, and threw a temper tantrum. She then grabbed me by the hair, dragged me to my bedroom, took off my clothes, tied me to the bed post, and locked the door.

Tom: Joe... you don't think that was at all abusive?

Dad: I guess I had never really thought about it that way.

Tom: Let's do an exercise. I'd like to rewrite history with you, Joe. I want you to picture yourself in that situation again, talking to your mom. Now, when she tries to grab you by your hair, I want you to visualize yourself shoving her back against the wall...HARD. In fact, you shove her so forcefully, that she hits her head against the wall and loses consciousness.

Now picture yourself frolicking all the way to the creek, smiling, enjoying the beautiful weather, and having fun with your friends, getting as dirty as you like. A couple of hours pass, and it is getting dark, so you head back home. Waiting for you in the yard is your mother, crouching down with open arms. You run to her and give her a great big hug. And then you apologize saying, "I'm sorry for hurting you, Mom." And picture her responding, "I forgive you Joe." And, now, turn to that little 9-year-old boy, Joe. Say to your 9-year-old self, "Joe, I will never let anyone hurt you again."

At that moment, my dad began to sob uncontrollably.

When I came home from a performance that evening, he was not wearing his Bi-PAP machine. He was sitting up straight, eating, smiling, and breathing on his own. He had transitioned his daytime usage of the breathing assist machine down from twelve hours to two. He made this transition over the course of the hour-long visualization exercise.

DAN WIONS

One last source of blessings in disguise that must be specially mentioned here is my daughter, Julie. Julie is a great source of joy in our lives. The playful, outgoing, innocent side to her personality serves up a constant stream of entertaining antics. She does her part to help around the house, is very affectionate, and makes sure that we know how much she appreciates all that we do for her. Julie is also a principled young person with a strong set of values that would make any parents proud and leave them feeling confident of her ability to lead a productive and meaningful life. In addition, she is a beautiful and exceptionally talented twenty-seven-year-old with aspirations of building a successful career as a model, actress, and business owner. You may be thinking: Every young woman is beautiful and talented in the eyes of her father. The truth is, in Julie's case, it is actually true.

As I have written earlier, it is also true that Julie has struggled with some serious neurological and emotional issues for most of her life. Like most young people, as Julie has grown from child to young adult, she has provided her mother and me with a great deal of joy, as well as numerous opportunities for personal and parental growth. While many of the difficulties we have experienced in rearing her reflect normal developmental patterns,

> Having a parent with a terminal illness challenged me to grow in ways I had never imagined. It challenged me to take down walls, to open up to the possibility of losing my father before I was ready...you're never ready. It challenged me to provide in certain ways I never thought I could, at that age especially. As overwhelming as that experience was, Dad still found ways to be my rock. I have fond memories kneeling by his wheelchair, laying my head on his heart and listening to it beat softly, as I'd hold his arms around me. He no longer had the strength to hold on to me himself. Yet, while he might not have been able to physically embrace me during my more vulnerable moments, I could feel his love shining through his weakness. He was still warm, steady, supportive and present, in his own way. I am so grateful to have had a father with that kind of capability; with that expansive capacity for love and nurturing.
>
> **JULIE WIONS**

her health issues have often magnified the intensity and tested our parenting abilities to their limits.

So how does all this tie in to a picture of Julie as a source of blessings in disguise? Well, as you can imagine, and may have experienced firsthand, raising a child with disabilities can be extremely stressful (come to think of it, raising any child can at times be extremely stressful). When I was diagnosed with ALS, it forced me to re-evaluate how I was dealing with that stress. As an illness in which the motor neurons become progressively compromised, excessive stress must be avoided wherever possible.

Like any parent, my children exhibit behaviors from time to time that run contrary to the way I would like to see them behave. In my more vulnerable and/or judgmental moments, I must admit to becoming irritated or even angry. With ALS, I could no longer afford the stress of these emotions. Through my experience with this illness, one of the things I have come to appreciate at a much deeper level is the understanding that when we are troubled by another person's behavior, it is often because that behavior reflects something in us with which we are not satisfied or comfortable. It is in this context that my beautiful and talented daughter emerges as one of my most potent sources of blessings in disguise.

In the process of applying what I had learned from Tom about living life in affirmation, I began to notice things about Julie's behavior that had escaped me for years. When Julie is feeling vulnerable, for example, she can quickly overreact to the most benign and mundane situation as if her life were being threatened. This, of course, is heightened by the anxiety that comes with having Tourette's. In response to a simple question about something like her schedule for the day, for example, I have observed her voice quickly increasing in intensity as if she were under duress. For years, I had tried—with limited success—to coach her through such moments, teaching her ways to manage stress and focus attention on defusing her sensitivity.

With an intensified commitment to managing my own stress, I began to notice that the behaviors of hers I found most disconcerting were behaviors I had been unconsciously modeling for her throughout her life. One day, as I was attempting to coach her through a rough moment, it hit me like a ton of bricks that I was modeling the very strained emotional reaction I was trying to coach her through with the irritated tone of my own voice. It is unclear to me whether Julie ever noticed a shift in my behavior stemming from that moment, but for me, it was an epiphany that forever changed my perspective and approach with her ... and myself.

This revelation was an extremely painful gift to receive. Yet, it has been one of the most powerful and healing experiences of my adventures with ALS. Julie pushes me to learn and grow, not just because she has struggles—we all do—but because she keeps bringing those struggles to me. After all, a child has at least as much difficulty with the parents' behavior as the parents do with the child's. While many children back away and even shut their parents out, Julie keeps coming back, even when my behavior has been less than supportive. She has become my mirror and unwitting mentor. She certainly lets me know when my behavior does not serve her well, but she also honors me by acknowledging how I have grown as a parent and why she keeps coming back for guidance and support. Each year, I am enamored by the increasing level of growth and confidence Julie displays in her formidable arsenal of skills and talents, especially in light of the emotional implications of coping with an ill parent. I remain grateful for the valuable contribution she makes to my ongoing evolution and healing through her own developmental adventures.

Fear and uncertainty are only natural under these types of conditions. But what makes Dad so remarkable is that through the darkness and the raging currents, he embraced and confronted these emotions. He chose to grow, to accept, and to learn. He chose to forgive, and to surrender to each moment, without giving up. He took on this challenge, for himself, and out of love for his family. He defines courage. He is my hero.

JULIE WIONS

CHAPTER EIGHTEEN

Human Will

and the Power of Choice

In my work as a management consultant, one issue that always proved to be a fertile ground for learning with my clients was the subject of "choice." Frequently, in the pursuit of improved business performance, executives discover that the unconscious choices they make about how to engage business issues and colleagues have a great deal to do with the results they achieve.

For example, it is quite common and appropriate for executives to hold employees accountable for meeting business objectives and to provide them feedback on their business-related behaviors and results—but frequently these same executives fail to examine how their own behaviors impact employees' success. Although it can be quite unnerving, consciously choosing and engaging in honest self-assessment often opens up huge growth opportunities for executives, their employees, and the business.

Helping people in business to clarify and become more accountable for the choices they make is a process that I had always found to be intriguing, rewarding, and enjoyable. In learning to deal with a life-threatening illness, however, I found myself once again in the role of student rather than mentor. While grappling with some of the most difficult decisions I'd ever known, I discovered a stronger connection between choice and will than I had ever faced in my professional endeavors.

Life and the media are filled with examples of people who have beaten the odds and overcome seemingly insurmountable obstacles through sheer force of will. What comes to mind is the absurd scene in *Monty Python and the Holy Grail* in which the Black Knight is trying to prevent Arthur from crossing a bridge. Each time Arthur relieves the knight of one of his appendages, the knight dismisses Arthur's success with some belittling comment. At one point during the fight, with blood gushing from his armless shoulder like water from a fire hydrant, the knight shouts, "Ah, it's only a flesh wound!" Finally, reduced to an armless and legless torso, the defiant knight screams after the departing Arthur, "Come back here, you lily-livered coward! I'll bite your knee caps off!" Despite the goriness of the scene, you have to admire the knight's tenacity. Each time I have lost a little more mobility, I have thought of the silly Black Knight, forever inspired by his refusal to quit.

Even more awe-inspiring because of their shocking reality are news stories of men who cut off their own arms in order to survive life-threatening accidents. Aron Ralston, a lone hiker whose arm had become wedged between two boulders after he fell into a crevasse, had to face the grim reality that he might die of starvation or exposure by the time anyone found him. His strong will to live enabled him to make—and carry out with—the impossible choice of severing his own arm to free himself. James Franco played Ralston in the movie, *127 Hours.*

Another story was of a farmer who was reported to have gotten his hand caught in a large piece of farm equipment that was quickly drawing him inside. He was left with only seconds to choose between having his entire body dragged into the gears of the machine or cutting off his own arm to survive. Like the hiker, the farmer somehow found the strength of will to separate mind from body long enough to perform the unthinkable.

Hollywood has produced numerous stories about people who have overcome enormous odds to achieve various kinds of success. The ones I find most inspiring are those that are based on true stories. One of my favorite examples is of Chris Gardner – played by Will Smith in *The Pursuit of Happyness.* Gardner, a determined and devoted father, overcomes his wife's desertion, theft, financial ruin, and homelessness to take care of his son and go on to achieve enormous financial success. Erin Gruwell—played by Hilary Swank in *Freedom Writers*—is a Los Angeles high school teacher who refuses to accept the failure of students on whom the system had given up. She invests long hours and her own money, sacrifices her marriage, exercises impressive creativity, and extends herself personally to build students' self-esteem and confidence. She even risks physical harm to overcome system resistance and achieve unprecedented success for her students.

Two more examples are even more directly relevant to my current situation. One is the story of Augusto and Michaela Odone – played by Nick Nolte and Susan Sarandon in the movie, *Lorenzo's Oil*—who put their careers on hold to find a cure for their son's life-threatening illness. They have to overcome financial obstacles as well as intense resistance, fear, and disbelief from both the medical community and parents of children facing the same disease. Refusing to accept their son's painful demise as inevitable, these two remarkable people are driven by their love for their child to achieve what the medical and pharmaceutical establishments had been unable to do: discover the cure that would save their child and many others.

Finally, Norman Cousins writes about recovering from a life threatening disease through the extensive use of humor, a positive attitude, and mega-Vitamin C therapy in his book, *Anatomy of an Illness as Perceived by the Patient: Reflections on Healing*. Cousins is yet another example of an individual who refused to accept the limits of conventional knowledge, took responsibility for his own destiny, and found a creative way to beat the odds and survive.

Each of these situations demonstrates the incredible power of the human will. It seems that the most important lesson is that the exercise of will is, in fact, a choice. All of these individuals chose to survive or succeed for themselves and/or for others. Every individual has that power.

And some use their power to make different types of choices than survival. In the 1981 film, *Whose Life Is It Anyway?* Richard Dreyfuss plays an artist who is totally paralyzed from the neck down following a car crash. Dreyfuss's character demonstrates an enormous amount of strength and determination in pushing the system relentlessly to allow him to act on his choice to die. Dr. Jack Kevorkian made a dark name for himself by supporting his patients in fighting that battle.

It is far too easy to categorize people who overcome larger-than-life circumstances as exceptional and heroic, while dismissing our own capacity to make similar choices. How many people do you know who constantly lament not having the "willpower" to lose weight, the energy to exercise regularly, or the initiative to find a job? Such issues are trivialized in the shadow of the stories above. We sell ourselves so short, so quickly.

The people in the stories above were average, everyday people just like you and me. What made them, their stories, and their results exceptional was their willingness to accept responsibility for their circumstances and outcomes. They each made conscious choices to pursue their desired results even in the face of tremendous challenge. Examples like these should make us all think harder about what we could achieve if we chose to be completely accountable for our actions and results.

I have spoken with and read about many other people who have been diagnosed with ALS. While some explore alternative ways of healing, others with whom I have spoken seem resigned to the fate dictated by the traditional medical paradigm. There are many who devote their time to fund-raising or have founded organizations devoted to accelerating the pursuit of a cure. Others continue to live their lives as fully as possible, finding creative ways to perform the work and activities they love despite their disability. Some choose to live out what they perceive as their final days with gusto, trying to make every precious minute count. Many live in fear of what they believe to be their inevitable demise, praying for the medical breakthrough that will save them from their fate. Still others sit in quiet desperation and depression, waiting for the end.

Steven Heywood devoted the last several years of his life with ALS working with his brother, Jamie, to establish a state-of-the-art research organization whose mission is to find and develop effective treatment and cure for this unforgiving disease. Steven has lost his battle with ALS, but the ALS Therapy Development Institute lives on as a testament to his will and his character. Augie Nieto, one of the most famous PALS (People with ALS) and author of *Augie's Quest*, has now risen to the challenge of using his formidable business skills to guide the institute's aggressive and relentless non-traditional research efforts in pursuit of a cure for ALS.

Ben Byer channeled his acting background into the production of *Indestructible,* the first feature-length documentary film about life with ALS. Regrettably, Ben lost his battle with ALS in July 2008, but his family is continuing the work of promoting his "indestructible" legacy. His film is winning critical acclaim in festival after festival. Steven, Augie, and Ben have all made courageous and inspiring choices about how to deal with their illness. Many others fight this illness in more private ways, yet they do so with a strength and courage that clearly reflects the power of their will.

The choice I have made about ALS is unusual, but not unique. I have chosen to relentlessly pursue the restoration of my nerves and muscles and heal my body. In his book, *Eric Is Winning*, Eric Edney shares his successes in pursuing recovery from ALS through alternative medical treatment to inspire hope.

I would not pass judgment on any of the different kinds of choices made by my ALS peers—or, for that matter, by people who struggle with their weight, their physical condition, or their career satisfaction. My sole intention here is to share some sources of inspiration in the hope that they will encourage others to accept responsibility for their choices and recognize opportunities to make bigger, more rewarding ones. When big issues arise, many of us do not hesitate to throw ourselves into the fight. But my warning is that, by not resolving smaller issues, many of us continue to carry around the stress of disappointment and dissatisfaction until it wears us down and makes us ill.

Even those who have chosen to succumb to a terminal illness without a fight still have choices to make about how to live out their final days. There are people with ALS who have withdrawn into themselves and are living out their last days in fear and anguish.

> "That's the thing, to keep going, manifesting your intention, even when things are really tough or uncomfortable. I mean, if you are going to break down when things are tough, that means you have a breaking point, a limit (hmm, even following my own advice as I speak). To ensure that one stays well, one basically has to have no breaking point and be unlimited and the more that this is true for a person, the more readily the person is going to succeed in changing things for the better."
>
> **MARTY MURRAY**
> **AUTHOR OF THE HEALING CHRONICLES BLOG.**

Others, while expecting the "inevitable," have chosen to embrace what life they have left with enthusiasm and gratitude. In so doing, they find that their quality of life is filled with more peace, pleasure, and comfort.

One of the many valuable gifts that have emerged from my life with ALS is a heightened awareness of human potential. We possess an astounding capacity to accomplish whatever is important to us. We also have the capacity to undermine and dismiss our true potential. What determines which capacity gets exercised is our willingness to make conscious, responsible decisions. I believe that we owe ourselves, and each other, our best possible choices, in all areas of our lives.

CHAPTER NINETEEN:
Shifting the Mindset

The many lessons of ALS have produced a shift in my thinking that has positively impacted my health as much as, if not more than, any treatment I have pursued. I have learned the importance of humor and joy, the power of surrender and affirmation, and how to find power in vulnerability.

My daughter once asked me, "Dad, what are your greatest fears?" I responded with two things: having a child with disabilities and being paralyzed. We both burst into a fit of laughter. Laughing at life's ironies and absurdities helps me shift more quickly to a positive mind-set when the threat of a dark moment looms. Since my diagnosis, there have been many of those!

For as long as I can remember, I have enjoyed observing and commenting on life's little absurdities. The practice has often come with a bit too much sarcasm at the expense of friends and family, but over the years, with Diane's help, I have gotten better at toning it down. I have also gotten better at picking appropriate partners with whom to exchange playful barbs. My sense of humor serves me well in fending off the stresses of living with ALS, and helps put others at ease who may feel awkward in the presence of someone who is physically impaired.

My favorite Joe activity (and one of his too, I believe) was taking him shopping at Lowes home center. Not only was it a road trip/change of scenery from the house, but also an opportunity to mess with the employees' heads. After we got the light bulbs and batteries, we would always go to the power tools and ladder sections and engage the employees in a discussion of which would be the best choice of chainsaw or 35' ladder for Joe to use. He and I would be ultra-serious—and the looks on the employee's faces were priceless. We had a lot of laughs in the van on the way home.

LEE SCHRAETER
FAMILY FRIEND

Since the 1960s, when Norman Cousins laughed himself back to health (as documented in *Anatomy of an Illness* starring Ed Asner), there has been a good deal of research on the effects of laughter and humor on well-being. Studies show that laughter yields the positive effects of reducing stress and pain, lowering blood pressure, and boosting the immune system. Knowing this, I incorporate as much joy, humor, and laughter as possible into each day.

Every day I make a conscious effort to focus my attention only on things that bring me joy and satisfaction. Rather than laboring over a task that is non-essential, I abort the activity. If a task is not particularly enjoyable but must be done, such as paying a bill, ordering supplies, or managing finances, I focus on the aspects of the activity that are satisfying and rewarding.

Diane and I enjoy watching movies together, and we often invite friends over to watch them with us. While we often watch comedy, we also enjoy action movies and dramas. When a film becomes a little bit too intense, my sense of humor kicks in to lighten the moment and draw a laugh out of a serious scene.

Another thing that brings me great joy is being outdoors. I have always been a lover of nature. No longer climbing mountains, skiing or diving, I still enjoy it in the simplest of contexts, whether watching wild animals frolic in the backyard, sitting out in the sun reading with Diane, taking long drives into the countryside, or visiting parks. Winters can be difficult since the cold weather takes a drastic toll on both my body and the availability of animals and foliage to observe. With spring and summer come greater freedom and opportunities to engage in more outdoor activities. Taking trips to the health food store, exploring local flower gardens, and visiting friends and family, we pack in as much outdoor activity as we can during the warmer months, especially when Diane is off from school.

In my more able-bodied days, I was a jogger. For the longest time, I found myself reluctant to join Diane for walks because, compared to jogging, they were boring. Eventually, out of desire to spend more quality time with my wife, I discovered the joy of sharing an hour walking with Diane to observe the local foliage and wildlife, take in the fresh air and smells of spring and summer, and most importantly, catch up on life. We continued this tradition for several years, even after the effects of ALS began to take their toll. As my legs lost more and more strength, I would reflect on those days of reluctance to walk rather than run. It made me laugh at myself to think how nice it would be to just be able to walk with a cane.

Eventually, walks were reduced to rolls in my wheelchair, with Diane pushing. The first wheelchair, a manual one, was a gift from our friends, Carol and Frank. The first time Diane and I attempted to use the chair was on one of our walks. As we prepared to leave the house, however, we discovered to our dismay that our friends had forgotten to provide the footrests for the chair. Undaunted and determined, we sat and pondered for a while how we could improvise. Sitting stationary in the wheelchair, my eyes darted around the garage searching for creative ideas on how to prevent my feet from dragging on the ground as Diane pushed me around the neighborhood. Finally, the image of my son's roller blades sitting up against the garage wall came into view, and, fortunately, we were the same shoe size.

Years earlier, on a Florida vacation, I had tried rollerblading with his skates, but I had proven to be a complete klutz at rollerblading from the normal upright position—the only things that saved me from a serious back injury were Dan's strong, waiting arms positioned protectively behind me in anticipation of a fall. But, as it turned out, wheelchair skating was much more manageable.

Soon after Diane and I began our walk, I discovered the advantages the skates provided. What had been impossible to do standing on the blades, was easy from the wheelchair. It took no time at all before I was steering us from side to side in a curving pattern down the street, as if carving my way down a ski slope. The subtle hills of our neighborhood provide exciting opportunities to free-style. Diane would let go of the wheelchair and I would cut a path down the road, changing the direction of the blades by tilting my knees from side to side. There was still enough strength in my legs to control the skates and even extend the heels to use the brakes. When we arrived at their house a few miles away to pick up the footrests, Carol and Frank were amused how I was steering the chair as Diane pushed me up their driveway.

Diane and I enjoyed our roller blade/wheelchair walks for several months. When my muscles atrophied to the point that a motorized vehicle was required, I had to find new ways to have fun. The motorized three-wheel scooter and, later, a power-wheelchair, both provided just enough speed to force Diane into a trot as I held her hand while driving the vehicle. Although she would beg me to let go, the occasional ploy reduced us both to frequent belly laughs. I was finally getting her to jog!

. . .

Of all the mental shifts with which I have had to wrestle, perhaps the most difficult has been acceptance of the need to surrender. This concept has been a source of significant struggle, and it is my strong suspicion that I am not alone in this regard. My friend and bodywork therapist, Nick, was probably the first person to guide me toward serious exploration of the meaning of surrender and its importance. Having battled a serious illness of his own, he had acknowledged that his healing did not begin until he had learned to surrender.

My initial reaction to his revelation was to recoil. "Surrender" sounded like giving up. Yet, here was someone whom I trusted telling me that he had survived a serious illness by giving up. It didn't make sense. I was truly confounded, and the fight in me triggered a surge of resistance that had to be constantly subdued in order to open myself to learning.

I am often troubled when I hear people lament about the inability to change. Dad was an example of someone who chose to change on multiple levels. You are reading about the fundamental shifts in his belief system, and about how grateful he was to everyone who helped accommodate his lifestyle adjustments. What he doesn't mention was his ability and willingness to change to accommodate people he loved.

The sound sensitivity my sister and I experienced from Tourette's Syndrome is called "Echolalia." To ease our suffering, Dad would completely change his speech patterns any time he was around us. He continued to do this even after the advanced stages of ALS made his talking laborious and unintelligible. Change is a choice. With the right motivation and guidance, anyone can accomplish it. Dad would much rather be remembered as someone who provided that type of empowering guidance, than as some lone miracle man who accomplished something few others could.

DAN WIONS

Working with affirmations—and one in particular—it finally hit me. The affirmation that brought it home was this: "I believe in living in the moment, total present time, going with the flow, and loving the challenges." After months of reciting this mantra daily, sometimes several times a day, it occurred to me what surrender really meant. And reading Eckhart Tolle's work, *The Power of Now*, helped to deepen my understanding of the concept. It finally became clear that *surrender* wasn't about giving up at all. It was simply about accepting the reality of the moment. It was about giving up resistance, not hope or intention. Prior to this revelation, I would allow fear to overtake me every time some lost level of strength suggested further progression of the disease.

For example, if I were having difficulty grasping my toothbrush, the terrifying thought would immediately crash into my brain, "Oh, my God, another basic daily task I can no longer do on my own." In truth, these minor losses have almost always proven to be temporary—and even when they haven't been temporary, panic has never been helpful. After learning to surrender during these moments, to stop resisting the immediate reality, the losses and the fear would quickly ease, if not dissolve. Sometimes I might even laugh at myself.

There are a number of things that can cause a temporary loss of strength or functionality: fatigue, gastrointestinal distress, the stress of pain or discomfort, or general stress, among them. Experience has taught me that the moment I allow myself to enter the realm of, "Oh, my God," instead of focusing on the simple reality—"At this moment I cannot brush my teeth"—the fear fuels stress and exacerbates my inability to move. Once I learned to surrender to the moment and not project it into the future as a symbol of something much worse, fears would dissolve, my body would relax, and strength would return. Often within seconds or, at most, a few minutes, I find enough strength in my hands to grasp the toothbrush and complete the job.

It takes considerable diligence to stay on the productive side of that fine line between surrender and resignation. To effectively surrender, I must stay in the moment and abandon all the judgments and projections that will invariably generate fear and doubt. The minute a connection is made between the current circumstances and past experience or future expectations, the moment opens up to a frightening array of negative emotions. The thought of a moment's weakness becoming a future trend assaults my emotions, which limits me physically and further fuels the fears I have created. These are the very same fears that most of us experience when we choose to resign ourselves to our "fate"—in other words, when we give up.

The classic image used in Gestalt psychology of a half-glass of water poses the eternal question: "is the glass half empty or half full?" When you choose to perceive the glass as half empty, you have chosen resignation. If you see it as half full, you have chosen to live your life affirmatively, and surrender becomes your weapon for fending off the scary moments when things don't appear to be going your way.

The person who has chosen resignation is constantly thinking and talking about all that is wrong or painful or dissatisfying in his life. He is constantly experiencing pain and discomfort—but ironically, the more he dwells on it, the more pain and discomfort he gets. By contrast, living in affirmation generates thoughts and conversation about all that is good and satisfying in one's life. It became clear in *The Secret* that *because* the person making this choice focuses consistently on all that he is grateful for (the glass half full), he attracts more of the same. Making this choice, I *expect* things to go well. So, when something painful or disappointing comes up, it appears merely as a momentary distraction on a positive path.

One time I needed feedback on my resume for a series of job interviews.... I wanted to ask Joe but I was so nervous about asking for help, about potentially burdening him when he had so much on his plate. I was so nervous I actually rehearsed asking him with the rest of the family! When nervous, I tend to laugh. So I was basically sitting in his office, laughing uncontrollably.... He was able to calm me down and assure me that it was okay to ask, and that he enjoyed helping and coaching people when he could.

Afterwards, I took a deep breath, and he just looked at me and exclaimed, "That was IT???!!!" We both chuckled.

Joe had that way about him. He made me feel so comfortable; I probably could have told him anything.

INNA KAPLAN
CLOSE FRIEND OF DAN

As such, it becomes easier to surrender to that moment and choose a life-affirming focus. This shift in mind-set has eliminated an enormous amount of stress from my life, replaced it with a healthy infusion of peace, and helped build the foundation for my healing.

• • •

When I became paralyzed, I found it all too easy to begin seeing myself as diminished and weakened. I started to think about all of the things I could no longer do, all of the opportunities that were no longer open to me. Playing tennis, going on vacations, earning a living, and even taking a walk with Diane all took on the form of fond, distant memories of a rich former life, with no place in the current or future reality. Even worse, I became dependent on others for the simplest activities of daily living. It was not difficult, in the context of such dramatic changes, to begin thinking of myself as weak, even powerless, and vulnerable. Compounding the situation was the awkward reaction of others who, while trying to hide their own discomfort and show compassion, found it difficult to disguise their pity and uneasiness.

Of course, the more I allowed this negative perspective and these reactions of pity to dominate my thoughts, the weaker and more vulnerable I became. While shifting to thinking in affirmation and gratitude, I have always been amazed to discover the constantly expanding power that can be born of vulnerability.

I cannot currently run around a tennis court or swing a racquet, but I can exercise with Therabands. I can also visualize myself playing tennis, programming my brain to repair the nerves and muscles that may make it possible to return to the tennis court in the future. While taking walks with Diane may not currently be an option, we can still be together and enjoy each other's company using the wheelchair. Handling the logistics and hectic demands of a management consultant—traveling, lecturing, facilitating, and coaching—are no longer within my present capabilities, but with creative use of the computer and the help of a friend, I can strive to inspire others to rise to their own challenges.

> I thought I was doing Joe this biiiiig favor. I'd "take care" of him for a month when I was between jobs. He's this nice guy, had a bad break in life. Boy, am I a nice person....
>
> Who would'a thought...I learned what a "nice person" really was! I learned what the word "survivor" really means. I learned how to care. How to give. How to ask for help. How to give back. How to make people feel important, doing the most menial of tasks.
>
> **MICHAELE DIVITO**
> LONGTIME FRIEND

So the first step to finding power in vulnerability has been to let go of opportunities lost, and focus on the different and new ones that my new circumstances have opened. I have become less prone to thinking, "I can't…" and more likely to ask, "How can I?" With this question comes a great deal of learning and creativity. In writing portions of this book, for example, I may exhaust myself typing with a mouse and an onscreen keyboard, but with the aid of voice software and friends, I am able to make much greater progress. This demonstrates the second step of finding power in vulnerability, which is to acknowledge and utilize your resources.

As mentioned earlier, it wasn't easy to ask for help at first. Even now, I find myself frequently testing the limits of the assistance I receive. I constantly check in with friends to ensure that my requests are reasonable, and assure them that others are available to pitch in if their plates are already full. To further ease these concerns, I often remind myself of the gift that people derive from giving and helping. Finally, I look for every opportunity to give back. I find a huge reward in using my professional skills to coach and teach others whenever the opportunity arises. By keeping fairness and exchange in mind, I more easily accept the help that others provide, and I accomplish far more than I ever thought my physical condition would allow.

Perhaps the most difficult issue in maintaining my power is dealing with the awkward and misguided approaches that others have in reaction to my vulnerable condition. About a year ago, I experienced a situation that exemplified how condescending and humiliating a well-intentioned person can be while acting on misguided assumptions. I was sitting in line at the supermarket checkout on a day when the weather permitted me to get out and run some errands with my aide.

196

An obviously well-meaning elderly woman sauntered up with a huge smile on her face and said, "Isn't it nice to get out?" I am quite certain that in her attempt to be compassionate and caring she was totally oblivious to the patronizing and condescending nature of her words and assumptions.

While a part of me found her behavior somewhat comical, it also triggered an angry flood of possible responses coursing through my brain: "How dare you assume that I am totally housebound?" or "How dare you assume that my life is so limited and shallow that a trip to the grocery store is such a huge event for me?" or "Is this something you would say to me if I were standing on two feet instead of being in a wheelchair, or would you simply say, 'Beautiful day, isn't it?'" "In fact, would you even be talking to me, a perfect stranger, if I were not sitting in this wheelchair?" Appreciating her kind intentions, however, I put my indignation aside and simply responded, "Yes, it's great being outside." I then proceeded to follow Lloyd through the checkout line, leaving the well-meaning stranger to her delusions.

Among the things that help me react to such situations without anger are the painful memories of foolish things that I have done in the presence of physically challenged individuals when I was able-bodied. A situation comes to mind from some thirty years ago in which I was making fun of a friend's oversized thumb while enjoying the hospitality of a woman who had been born deformed by Thalidomide. There I was, wagging my friend's thumb around in a perverse and bizarre attempt at humor to break up an awkward pause in conversation, as our hostess, whose upper body appendages consisted of a total of five fingers growing out of her two shoulders, sat and watched in quiet consternation.

As we said our goodbyes and drove away from the house, my wife and friends did not waste time in sharing how mortified they were by my insensitive behavior. It was only at that point that it began to dawn on me the horrible thing I had done. I had known our hostess long enough to know that she had very strong feelings about being treated like anyone else. I had also been aware for some time of my feelings of awkwardness, discomfort and ignorance about how to behave appropriately in her presence. Until that moment, the depth of these feelings had not been clear to me. I was too immature and humiliated to know how to phrase an apology, even if I had had the courage to turn around and attempt one. More than three decades later, my gut still wrenches at the thought of this episode. That I never created the opportunity to make things right is one of my greatest regrets.

As someone who is now the occasional recipient of such awkward behavior, I always try to respond with compassion and good humor. So now, when someone standing five feet away quietly asks my wife, "So how is Joe doing?" I will playfully shout out, "I'm doing great. How are you?" demonstrating that I am perfectly capable of carrying on the conversation myself. Or when someone, meeting me for the first time, fidgets with his hands wondering how to greet a person who can't move his, I will quip, "I'd love to shake your hand, but you'll have to do the work, so pick one and have at it." Openly playing with the awkwardness my disability creates is a great power. It relieves the tension, gently reminds people that I am still a person, not a disease, and helps us both avoid embarassment.

CHAPTER TWENTY:
Living in Affirmation
Despite Evidence to the Contrary

While the results can be incredibly rewarding, shifting the way you think is both a fascinating and a difficult process. From 2002 to 2006, I watched my body being eaten away from the inside out. The experience often seemed surreal. At times, I felt like a detached observer, staring in consternation as my muscles melted away, leaving my skeletal frame more and more exposed through my sagging skin. In those moments when it struck me that it was actually *my* body that was disappearing before my eyes, emotions like terror, anger, confusion, frustration, depression, and defiance would flood me with crushing force.

By the end of 2006, building on what I had learned from Tom, Tamara, and Sue, I was beginning to shift away from a mentality of defying and avoiding death to one of valuing and rebuilding my life. With that shift came increasingly frequent positive emotions like hope, determination, peace, resolve, gratitude, and confidence. But, when the person staring back at you from the mirror is barely more than half your normal weight and lacks the strength to hold or move a pencil or even wiggle a toe, belief in recovery can be difficult to maintain. Instead, doubt and skepticism became my most persistent assailants. I had to constantly remind myself that whether or not the physical evidence supported my intention to recover, the only chance I had was to strengthen my belief that it was possible. The choice had become simple:

> Joe, you are the man of miracles. No one could ever imagine the battle you have waged for all these years. You are a hero to all of us. Your will to live and to strategize against the evil giant mirrors a David and Goliath of our time. You are an inspiration to all of us.
>
> **JUDI NICKELSON**
> LONGTIME FRIEND

believe, as the doctors had told me, that there is no recovery from ALS and death, or believe that recovery is possible and discover how to do it. I had nothing to lose and everything to gain by believing in healing.

Once Tom and Tamara enabled me to see how I was literally thinking myself to death, the objective became clear. I had to start thinking as a living person who expected to go on living. Easy to say. Yet, while still evolving in the ability to do this, it feels as if I am largely there. For example, when thinking about the future, I now envision myself in a more mobile body, participating in activities I enjoyed before becoming paralyzed. I plan my weeks to be productive and enjoyable, doing things that bring a sense of accomplishment and satisfaction. This is a far cry from the fear, despair, and desperation I felt in the earlier stages of my illness. What seems most amazing to me is my ability to stay on this positive path even as my body has continued to show signs of deterioration.

So how do I maintain a sense of conviction and belief in recovery in the face of evidence to the contrary? Am I simply delusional, or have I created a reality that supports my intention? By accepting vulnerability, I find so much more power in the capabilities I still have, and more pleasure in allowing others to assist me. To get to a point where I could routinely, and almost instinctively, apply these concepts in my daily life, required four things: a strong conviction, an ability to temporarily suspend belief, some structure, and a paradigm shift. While the importance of a strong conviction may seem obvious, the maintenance of it is not. It took a deliberate and focused effort to suspend certain beliefs, incorporate supportive structures into my daily practices, and open myself to the full possibilities of alternative medicine.

Suspension of belief actually had a double focus. On the one hand, I had to stop believing that imminent death was unavoidable. On the other hand, I had to stop doubting that I was getting better. Achieving this mental leap, however, only required a single strategy: the decision that focusing on death was not going to help avoid it. Moreover, I came to realize that, by thinking about a premature death, the Law of Attraction was operating to ensure that outcome. To obsess over the absence of physical evidence of improvements would activate the Law of Attraction in manifesting that undesirable image. Realizing that my only hope was to behave and think as if recovery was already under way, I began to structure my day to focus my thinking on the reality I was determined to create.

Step one was to create a written gratitude list. Since August 2006, when I began this process, I have religiously recited this list at the beginning of each day. The list consists of some obvious things and many others that we sometimes take for granted. I include things like the sky, the trees, the shrubs and the grass, the sun, the moon, the stars and the clouds. I also remind myself how grateful I am for the acrobatic hummingbirds, squirrels, and other wildlife that entertain me each day as they parade across the backyard by my window.

With great attention to their attributes, I acknowledge how grateful I am for my wife and children and the joy and growth they bring me. Also included in the list is an appreciation of my education, skills, and knowledge, and of all the people who support me in the effort to regain total health and mobility, and in my life in general. As the list has grown, I have found it important to allow the detail and scope of its content to evolve. It keeps me focused on the good in life, because I truly feel blessed by each and every element that I recite. Reciting the list is a very real and moving experience, with an almost prayer-like quality that begins each day.

The second structure that has enabled me to suspend and shift my beliefs is a written and then memorized list of affirmations, which I recite each morning, following the gratitude list. Over the past three years, my affirmations list has grown to about forty statements. In addition to saying them in the morning, I use some of these affirmative statements occasionally throughout the day. For example, if my fingers seem weaker at a given moment, I may invoke an affirmation such as, "I am safe and secure. I trust the process of life." This enables me to surrender to the moment and stay focused on what I have, rather than losing myself in the fear of what may have been lost. When someone else's behavior elicits feelings of anger or frustration, I recite the affirmation, "I have abundant energy, both creative and physical, to change my attitude and accept others as they are." This affirmation helps refocus my attention on the power I possess to accept and exercise responsibility for my thoughts and behavior, rather than blaming the other person for causing stress, and feeling powerless.

The final step that has helped me remain living in affirmation involves the acceptance of, and focus on, the paradigm of alternative medicine. In traditional western medicine, there is little treatment and no cure for ALS. By contrast, alternative medicine holds that *the human body always has the capacity to heal itself regardless of the diagnosis.* After months of practicing my gratitude list and affirmations, I was ready to replace the effort of suspending beliefs regarding my ultimate demise with creating new beliefs based on my body's capacity to heal. The more I focus on gratitude and affirmation, the more I come to believe in the certainty of recovery. The stronger this belief grows, the more I experience positive changes in my physical, emotional, and mental state. It took two years of practicing gratitude and affirmation to shift from suspended belief to true expectation of recovery.

Despite my stubbornness, I am not sure I could have maintained the strength of conviction to find a formula for healing without the embrace of my army of friends and relatives. As a result of their support, strength of will and conviction, and my willingness to recite affirmations even before I really believed them, the situation has evolved to the point where I am truly convinced of the reality of recovery. My health is far stronger than when I began this process in late 2006—I have fewer bouts of fatigue and coughing, much less pain, greater functioning and best of all, more energy to write this book! By all measures, the progression of the disease since then has been negligible. While doctors might attribute this to the unpredictability of ALS, I am convinced that the reason I am still alive and in better shape is a direct result of the mental shift I achieved and the actions I have taken because of it.

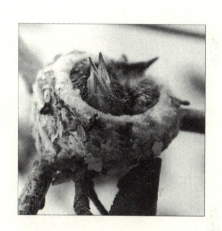

Part IV:

The Current Reality

JOSEPH L. WIONS

CHAPTER TWENTY-ONE:

A Typical Day

As soon as the first daylight pierces my eyelids and the cobwebs of sleep begin to clear from my brain, my attention turns to my forty affirmations, the recitation of which takes about 15 to 20 minutes. I acknowledge and appreciate the things I love and cherish in nature, in the people I value, and the functions of my mind, heart, body, and soul.

As a part of my morning affirmations, I play golf, baseball, tennis, ski, swim, hike, go rock climbing, and do other activities in my mind. By doing so, I believe that I am programming my brain to repair the nerve and muscle damage that currently prohibits me from enjoying these activities with my body.

I often complete my affirmations by 6:30 or 7:30, when my aide, Jimmy, cheerfully enters the room with a "good morning," and a "how are you?" If I have not yet finished my affirmations, he respectfully proceeds with the process of preparing me for the day as I continue. He begins with emptying the urinal and taking a fresh specimen from which to test my pH (which is how I keep track of the effects of diet on maintaining an alkaline system, in order to keep bacteria and viruses under control).

Next, he prepares some warm water, which I always try to drink early to encourage the desired bowel behavior later in the morning. Three mornings a week, the warm water is replaced by a maintenance dose of MMS (Miracle Mineral Solution) in apple juice and distilled water, to keep any pathogens to a minimum. Then, Jimmy carefully and thoroughly removes the stubble from my face, neck, and ears with my electric razor. After that, he rearranges the sheets and covers to keep me warm as we engage in the range-of-motion exercises that have evolved over the years: pushing, pulling, lifting, stretching, and rotating various body parts. Some of these motions are quite passive, and others require significant effort on my part. Consistent use of these exercises over the years has helped eliminate and prevent the return of joint pain, and has helped prevent and/or limit the stiffness and rigidity that can accompany the progression of ALS.

Often, as Jimmy takes me through some of the more passive exercises, like rotating my straightened arms in a circle from the shoulder, I find myself studying the detailed and taut appearance of his trim and well-defined musculature. It reminds me of what my own limbs used to look like. Watching his muscles flex as he takes my arms through their paces elicits visions of my own arms moving once again. I close my eyes and sink into that vision, enjoying the sensation of the movement and anticipating the day when I'll again be able to complete these exercises independently.

It usually takes about half an hour to complete the routine. This is followed by another half hour on the swing machine to get the blood flowing more actively in my legs. While the swing machine gently rocks my feet from side to side, Jimmy leaves the room to tend to other housekeeping chores. I use the quiet alone-time to engage in meditative exercises and prayer as the machine completes its work.

After the swing machine, it's time to get out of bed. Jimmy detaches the Bi-PAP from its humidifier, which keeps me from getting too dried out during sleep. He pulls back the covers, gently cradles my legs and shoulders, then turns and positions me into a sitting position on the edge of the bed. Placing his hands securely under my thighs and locking my knees with his to prevent sliding, he rotates me 90 degrees from the bed to the wheelchair. After a few attentive adjustments of legs, hips, head and shoulders (remember, I can *feel* everything; I just can't *move* well), he covers me with a warm blanket, and carefully places my right hand on the joystick that controls the wheelchair. I then position myself beside the bedroom bay window where I sit alone for the next fifteen minutes or so, dividing my attention between the news on TV and the antics of the birds and animals, while Jimmy prepares breakfast.

The grace, beauty and color of our backyard deer, squirrels, rabbits and birds always bring me delight. Squirrels, however, give something more. Incredibly resourceful and determined, these creatures certainly entertain. With their unparalleled persistence, they have managed to circumvent almost every obstacle thrown at them to discourage their invasion of my bird feeders. My latest attempt to subdue their voracious appetites is a device that spins the feeder in circles when the motor is activated by the squirrel's weight. The first time I watched one of these furry grey intruders clinging to the spinning feeder until he was thrown to the ground, I nearly hurt myself laughing. I watch the feeder each morning, hoping for another amusing attempt by the little thieves. Their comic perseverance inspires my own quest for renewal.

When Jimmy returns with my morning smoothie, it takes me ten or fifteen minutes to suck the breakfast mixture down through a straw, along with any supplement capsules with which I may be experimenting. The time it takes to consume a meal varies with the number of times a morsel of food or liquid sneaks past my weakened epiglottis, producing a coughing/choking episode in my body's attempt to clear the irritation in my trachea. This usually occurs at least once at every meal. Typically, these episodes last only a few minutes, but sometimes they go on for quite a while and require the use of a cough-assist machine to suck out the errant food particles. Prior to my work with José, the healer, these episodes often lasted for several hours. One of José's greatest contributions to my well-being has been a dramatic reduction in the frequency and duration of these coughing/choking fits.

Next come the bathroom activities, which usually begin with brushing my teeth. Jimmy places my hands on a folded towel at the edge of the sink, leans me forward to a balanced position, removes the Bi-PAP, and places the head of the electric toothbrush in my mouth. With the base of it between my overlapped hands, I spend about two minutes pushing the towel back and forth across the edge of the counter and using my tongue to rotate the toothbrush to make sure I polish every nook and cranny. This is one of the most physically demanding activities of a typical day. If I am not balanced just right, the process leaves me red in the face, out of air and exhausted, or in danger of falling forward and jamming the toothbrush down my throat.

From the sink, we move to the toilet, where Jimmy carefully positions me on an adaptive seat. He props me up with pillows to facilitate my balance and to ensure that I don't fall off. The slightest imbalance causes my muscles to work harder at keeping me in place, diverting much-needed energy from, you know, the task at hand. He also covers me with a blanket and points an electric heater at me to keep my ALS-diminished frame from getting too cold. During the moments on the throne, I often find myself thinking about Morrie Schwartz (*Tuesdays with Morrie*). In the book, he talks about his anticipation of reaching a point in the progression of his ALS where he would no longer be able to wipe his own butt. He described it as a kind of final step in the loss of dignity. My own experience of having reached that moment has been somewhat different. I find myself immersed in feelings of extreme gratitude that there are people in my life who willingly complete that task for me. While elimination is not always easy, I am very grateful that I still retain control of most bowel and bladder functions.

The next transfer is from the toilet to a padded shower seat. Jimmy positions me on the seat to ensure that my head, back, butt, and arms are aligned for comfort and balance, and then wheels it into position inside the shower stall. He hoses me down with a hand-held showerhead while scrubbing me with washcloths, dries me off, and places me back in the wheelchair. I often find myself marveling at how adeptly this 150-pound man safely transfers me so many times in a given day without injuring either of us. Several larger men who have preceded him in this job had to give it up because of back problems. I truly admire Jimmy's sense of pride in the work. Never content with his technique, he is always looking for ways to improve it.

Cleaned, dried, and blanketed for warmth, I am then helped back to the area between the bay window and the bed for dressing. After putting on my tee shirt and socks, and pulling underwear and pants up to my thighs, Jimmy lowers the footrest of the chair and tilts the chair forward in preparation for a much more delicate operation, the final and most difficult lift of the morning. While lifting me for transfer to another seat is not an easy procedure, the lift for dressing is a much more delicate operation.

In order to keep me standing, Jimmy must keep his knee securely pressed against mine to prevent my leg from buckling; he has to keep my left arm (the stronger of the two) hooked around his right shoulder, and maintain firm but gentle pressure on the small of my back to ensure that my body does not jack-knife backwards. While staying constantly focused on these three parts of my body, he has to reach down with his free hand and pull up my pants. If he were to lose focus for even a moment, a shift in position could cause me to drop like a stone. Jimmy has become masterful at managing this circus-like balancing act.

Many people with my level of paralysis use various forms of lifts, such as the Hoyer lift, to facilitate the transfers and dressing issues. Unfortunately, I have found these devices to be unbearably uncomfortable, cumbersome, and dehumanizing. I am very grateful to have consistently found aides who have been capable of moving me around manually. Touch also keeps a person feeling human.

On a good day, when everything runs smoothly, we will have exhausted about three and a half hours completing the tasks that would take a healthy person less than an hour. The fact that it takes *only* three and a half hours is a credit to Jimmy's adeptness—with some of his predecessors, the same activities took five hours or more.

By 10 or 11 o'clock in the morning, I am usually in my office, where I can access the computer. Since the dietary and psychological shifts I achieved two to three years ago, my energy levels enable me to spend significantly more time on the computer than I could four or five years ago, when I actually had greater use of my hands and arms!

I cannot imagine life without the computer. Now *this* machine affords a level of independence and productivity that would otherwise be absolutely unattainable. During the colder months, when it is more difficult to get outside, it is my portal to the world and insurance against isolation. The computer minimizes my dependency on others for a variety of needs. Instead of worrying about subjecting my body to the weakening effects of the cold, I simply go online and take care of most shopping needs without ever leaving the house. Through the computer, I can also make phone calls without having an aide standing by my side and holding the phone to my ear. When I can't reach people by phone, I can use e-mails to keep in touch.

Much of what I have learned from living with ALS and working at recovering has also evolved through the use of the computer. Internet search engines give access to just about anything in the world. Having been around long enough to experience the evolution from a paper-and-pencil world to a digital one, I live every day in awe of the access we have to information and each other. Between my network of friends and supporters and the Internet, I am constantly researching new possibilities to enhance my chances of success in beating this illness. With the computer, an on-screen keyboard, and the support of my "nimble-fingered friends" and family, I have managed to stay engaged with the world and people I know and care about.

By 12 or 12:30 in the afternoon, Jimmy will saunter into the office, requesting an order for lunch. As he prepares the meal, I usually place the first of my two daily phone calls to José, while continuing to check e-mail and work on my to-do list. I have always had a tendency toward multi-tasking, and reduced mobility doesn't appear to have changed that.

Conversations with José, the Healer, usually begin with a review of how well my arm strength is holding up, an assessment of breathing and swallowing for the morning, a report on my bowel movement, the pH level of my urine sample, and any other pertinent issues about how the body is functioning. If I notice and communicate any particular issues, like weakness in my hands or excessive itching in a sensitive area, he will begin by focusing his attention on that area of the body to intuitively determine the issue and resolve it. To begin the examination, he will launch into his mantra of, "right switch, left switch…" I have no idea what he is doing, but at the end of it he offers explanations of how he found poisons, toxins, crystallizations, or lack of communication between body parts, which were responsible for any difficulties reported. Along with these explanations, he also reports his degree of success in removing any undesirable substances or improving communication or functioning within my body. To the uninitiated or skeptical, this may all sound like a bunch of hooey. To be honest, I sometimes have my doubts. Yet, the improvements I have experienced in swallowing, air flow in the lungs, and the elimination or reduction of skin sensitivities since engaging with José are measurable—and a relief. Since my role in conversations with José is largely passive, I often eat lunch, and continue working on the computer while he completes his work. Lunch typically consists of a banana smoothie and a small salad of fruit and vegetables and hard-boiled eggs or sardines. Eggs and sardines are among the limited animal products I eat with any regularity. I include these through the guidance of Dr. David Perlmutter, author of *The Better Brain Book*. Perlmutter is a neurologist with significant experience in the treatment of neuro-degenerative diseases like MS, Parkinson's, and ALS. In his experience, these foods are rich sources of omega-3 and omega-6 oils, which the brain requires for optimal functioning.

In addition to work on the computer, weekday afternoons also routinely include about an hour of exercise. With assistance, I spend about fifteen minutes being bounced on a small trampoline, another ten minutes or so leaning forward and backwards for several dozen repetitions of a sit-up-like motion and completing a series of arm and leg exercises designed by José to encourage increased mobility. Beyond these routine activities, any given afternoon may include visits from friends, shopping excursions, acupuncture or other medical appointments, "walks" around the neighborhood, or other outings. During the warmer months, I especially look forward to walks with Diane.

Evenings begin with dinner, which typically consists of another smoothie and a larger salad. I pick dinner ingredients of fruits,

> As Dad wrote this book, he occasionally found himself excusing or defending certain aspects of his learning and healing process, or at least rationalizing for people who might not take some of these things at face value.
>
> The reality is, if he hadn't been sick, he probably would have dismissed the merit of many of these approaches. The thing to remember about such types of spiritual, metaphysical, and psychological work that Dad pursued is that they must be tailored to resonate with you. Using affirmations as an example, I personally resisted this approach for a long time, partly because I wasn't ready to examine myself that deeply, and partly because I found many of the affirmations to be a bit hokey. Once I found wording that resonated with me, though, affirmations had a profound impact on my life as well.
>
> **DAN WIONS**

vegetables, and herbs carefully for flavor and texture, since I use few spices (which are dehydrating) and no dressings (which add processed sugars and fat). While Jimmy prepares the evening meal, I complete some additional meditations and watch a little comedy on TV.

Dinner is often followed by more visitors, occasional shopping runs, excursions to Diane's concerts, more TV, or reading. Somewhere between 8:30 and 9:30 I usually make use of the swing machine again anywhere from twenty to ninety minutes. The machine seems to speed my digestive process (especially when I've had a little too much for dinner), and removes any discomfort from my legs in preparation for sleep.

Getting ready for bed involves a series of activities that take about forty-five minutes to complete. It begins with the tooth brushing ritual, followed by a brushing of my scalp. This brushing serves to massage the skin and stimulate blood flow, resulting in a reduced occurrence of scalp itching, which can sometimes interrupt sleep.

At this point, I am ready to be moved into bed. Once again, Jimmy grabs me under the arms, locks my knees with his own, sits back on his haunches, and swings me onto the edge of the bed. Next, placing one arm under my knees and the other behind my shoulders, he rotates me on my behind to position me on the bed. Before settling into a sleeping position, I am rolled onto my side for the application of a homeopathic salve to prevent itching and irritation in my private areas and tailbone from interrupting my sleep.

Once on my back and centered on the bed, Jimmy places folded towels under my hips to elevate the tailbone from the mattress. This prevents pressure pain from waking me in the middle of the night, since I cannot roll or shift easily. He also arranges some small pillows under my ankles to avoid pressure pain on my heels. After the evening phone chat with José, Jimmy can finally complete pulling up the sheets and blankets. He then places the urinal bottle between my legs so hopefully I can get through the night without disturbing Diane. One more check on the positioning of the Bi-PAP face mask to ensure comfort and a snug fit, some final adjustments to the pillow, blankets and bed, and I am at last ready for sleep.

I often reminisce over the days when I could strip off my own clothes, brush my teeth, and curl up on my side under the covers, all in ten minutes or less. Sleeping on my side is an experience that I can now enjoy for no more than twenty or thirty minutes before the constriction of my lungs and pressure pains on my shoulder and side rob me of the pleasure. Since the re-centering of my hips and the repositioning of pillows and towels would then fall on Diane's shoulders, it is a treat that I rarely seek in the middle of the night.

So, lying there on my back, ensconced in my elaborate arrangement of pillows and towels, almost completely immobile except for limited movement of my forearms and very narrow lateral motion of my head on the pillow, I count my blessings. I give thanks that I have adjusted to sleeping in this position, that I have a wonderfully supportive and efficient aide to take me through the bedtime process, and that the chronic pains and skin irritations that used to interrupt my sleep several times each night have been eliminated.

Then I sense Diane lying next to me. I long to roll over on my side, reach out to stroke her hair, massage her back, and make love to her. I struggle to resist wallowing in the frustrations over what I cannot do. To do so would be both mind- and gut-wrenching beyond imagination. Instead, I bring my memories into the present and enjoy the sensations in my mind that I cannot currently enjoy with my body. I let these thoughts shape and color my dreams of a reality that currently eludes me, yet motivates me to persist in my intention to heal.

On evenings when fatigue doesn't interfere, Diane will roll over and gently run her hand across my chest, face, neck and shoulders as we tenderly exchange kisses, restoring a small remnant of the physical reality we once shared.

It seldom takes me more than a few minutes to drift off to sleep. If I have trouble doing so, a meditation will help to resolve it quickly. In my dreams, I am almost always fully mobile or in

> Even with the devastation ALS caused, beautiful moments embraced our family. Not every day held darkness. In fact, most days shined with an array of love and optimism, as ALS became "normal." Our struggle painted a canvas of rich colors, despite a palette of gray.
>
> **JULIE WIONS**

the process of regaining my mobility. I believe that this is a reflection of my intention to heal.

My usual time in bed is actually shorter now than it was four or five years ago, due to an improved sleep pattern. Thanks to improvement in my diet, psychological orientation, and care, I typically sleep for about seven hours and rarely wake up more than once each night to pee. The diet and my outlook provide enough energy to get through the day productively and usually without fatigue. I rarely feel the need to nap any more. The efficient care from my health aides allows for an earlier start to the day. A full night's sleep and I'm ready to take on the world again, spending six to eight rich and fulfilling hours working at my new job: living, learning, and helping others with ALS.

CHAPTER TWENTY-TWO:

A Formula for Success

What is Working for Me

I do not claim to be an expert on recovering from ALS. Nor am I
qualified to offer medical advice. All I can offer is my personal
experience in the hope that others may find something in it that will
help in their own life journey. My readers will have to judge, based on
my results, if what I suggest for battling ALS (or any other difficult
challenge) makes sense to them and is worth the effort.

The first thing I had to address when facing the dreaded diagnosis
was whether I truly wanted to live, and how much. In spite of my
positive attitude, it really wasn't until three years after my diagnosis
when Tom Woloshyn came into my life, that I truly began to
consciously explore this issue. One of the first things he asked me was,
"Do you want to live or do you want to die?" I was startled. Wasn't it
obvious? But confronted with Tom's question, I had to ask myself to
what lengths I was willing to go. Suddenly it became clear that my
potential for success was highly dependent on what I really believed
and was actually committed to. As I discussed in Chapter 18, human
beings are capable of accomplishing the incredible, if not the
impossible, when they truly believe in the possibility of their goals and
are fully committed to achieving them.

I spoke earlier about how the very concept of "trying" implies the
possibility of failure. People who smoke or take drugs often claim they
are "trying" to stop; those who quit just do it. This is why it is so
difficult to break an entrenched habit. We can become as addicted to
our thoughts, beliefs, and appetites as we can to a drug. The latter part
of the film, *What the Bleep Do We Know?* offers a rather entertaining
cartoon animation that provides a more scientific explanation of this
phenomenon. The film describes how neural patterns that repeatedly

trigger our cravings and expectations are formed in the brain. While these patterns can be altered or replaced, it takes a deep commitment and hard work to do so.

From Tom and Tamara I had learned that I had become addicted to a thought process that was not supportive of healing. The conscious choice that I made to change it has pitted me against all conventional wisdom, which insists that escaping death from ALS is not only unrealistic, but impossible. The diminished capacity of my body frequently undermines the shift to a thinking pattern that will support recovery. To be successful, I must be extremely intentional and approach the task with a level of intensity and resolve that assumes no other possible outcome. There can be no equivocation. Of course there are frequent physical failures that test my resolve and cause me to waver, but when this occurs, I no longer "try" to believe. I remind myself to be responsible and accountable for my response.

When I now encounter pain or discomfort, doubt or fear, I do my best to tolerate it and focus on something productive or positive. When I encounter inconvenience, rather than wasting time lamenting over it, I shift my thoughts as quickly as possible to ways of either dealing with it or working around it. So when my hand won't turn the control stick on the wheelchair to the right, for example, I simply refuse to dwell on the fear that more strength may have been lost. Instead, I breathe, and focus on the movement that is still possible, and shift (with the help of an aide) to a position from which the turn is more negotiable, *all the while maintaining belief in my recovery with absolute conviction.* In this way, I work at breaking the negative thoughts and expectations to which I have become addicted, and replacing them with beliefs that support my goal.

Don't get me wrong—fear and doubt can be intimidating, and the goal can seem impossible to achieve. But now, moments of doubt are often followed by brief moments of disappointment that I've given in to doubt (which is actually quite different from getting stuck in doubt). Some of the hardest moments for me are when it seems like no one else can understand. During these moments, I feel alarmingly alone. To avoid getting lost in the grip of this particular negative thought process, I have learned to turn to an affirmation like, "I accept the abundance of healing energy in the universe, and I am grateful to participate" or "I believe I am healthy and balanced of mind, heart, body, and soul." When I'm in the middle of a coughing spell, or exhausting every ounce of strength trying to move my foot a sixteenth of an inch, words like these can be hard to believe. But by training myself to repeat affirmations until my thoughts are focused back on my belief in recovery, I have reached the point where the negative thoughts rarely last more than a few seconds.

Our social programming has taught us that when a doctor says it's over, it's over. Recovery becomes an impossible dream. Faced with the choice of accepting a premature and ugly demise versus believing in the possibilities of an alternative paradigm, though, it has not been difficult for me to go beyond the traditional medical model and set a goal for recovery. While the traditional medical paradigm offers no cure or effective treatment for ALS, there are always possibilities in alternative medicine. For someone with a strong will to live, this is not a difficult intellectual leap.

Learning to believe in the certainty of recovery is another story. It requires constant vigilance to achieve and maintain that belief. I truly hope that stem cell or genomics studies or some other medical research will someday produce a cure, and I do what I can financially and politically to support those efforts. But I have no intention of becoming another ALS statistic while waiting for that to happen. And so far, so good.

I strongly believe in the power of the human brain to alter bodily functions. I also believe we have the capacity to train our brains (i.e., alter our addictions) so that neural messages that will encourage healing can be sent to damaged cells. I have read from several sources that all the cells of the human body periodically replace themselves. If this is true, then why should it not be possible to replace damaged cells with healthy ones? This makes sense to me, yet my moments of doubt trigger fears that it may not happen. I can tell myself over and over again that I am going to beat this disease, but my gut is quick to remind me that I have not yet overcome my addiction to the fear of failure. I believe the key to recovery is buried in this constant internal struggle. The goal is to convince my mind so thoroughly of the certainty of recovery that my brain will consistently signal damaged nerve and muscle tissue to replace itself with healthy cells.

Each time a moment of doubt occurs, it reminds me of the healing work that remains towards reaching my goal. This nudges me to reflect on the progress already made, and to repeat affirmations until I am refocused on my intention, trusting the Law of Attraction to pull me back on track again. The alternative is to indulge the fears and allow my addictions to draw me closer to death. My intention to live must be reaffirmed again and again. There can be no excuses and no abdication of responsibility. Medical doctors and alternative practitioners can help, but I must always remember that my life and body are my responsibility and that I am always the primary and final decision-maker about my care.

. . .

Once I established an intention to recover and accept responsibility for achieving my goal, the rest of my program for healing became relatively easy to implement. After experimenting with dietary changes, dozens and dozens of vitamins and supplements, exotic forms of electronic equipment with purported healing properties, healing stones and medallions, and numerous other healing strategies, I have concluded that the rest of the healing process involves four things: *detoxification, optimal nutrition, exercise,* and *attracting healing energy.*

Detoxification

Detoxification, I have come to believe, is a critical issue for anyone residing on planet Earth. There is no escaping the fact that the human race has done an extensive job of polluting the planet's air, water, and soil. We all have a responsibility in stopping the destruction of our home and in creating a greener, more life-sustaining environment. As someone whose health is already severely compromised and vulnerable to the caustic effects of the current environment, I have a responsibility to protect myself from its ill effects. It is impossible to avoid exposure completely, so it is imperative to find effective measures for cleansing on a regular basis.

Our government supplies us with scientifically derived numbers regarding the acceptable parts per million of particulates in the air we breathe, the water we drink, and the food we eat. It also establishes standards to which food and pharmaceutical companies are held accountable for the safety of the additives and chemicals in their products. Yet, year after year, the news media blast us with stories about adverse reactions to drugs that kill people, the health risks associated with food dyes, bad fats, excessive salt and sugar in processed and fast foods. And, year after year, we ignore the warnings, choosing convenience over health. We continue to spray pesticides on our foods, process everything, tolerate the smokestacks and car fumes in our communities, and delude ourselves into thinking that our water is safe because we drink it from bottles. We ignore the warnings until we get sick. Then we search for the "right" doctor, who will give us a magic pill to make us feel better.

In doing so, we are abdicating responsibility for keeping our bodies clean and healthy as we further pollute them with the toxins inherent in most pharmaceutical products. I am not suggesting that we should abandon modern Western medicine and all pharmaceutical products in our attempt to preserve health or fight illness. These things have a place in maintaining and restoring health. I myself worked for a pharmeceutical company for years and believed in what I was doing. However, as a culture we are not educating and managing ourselves in ways that maintain healthy lives and a healthy environment.

Detoxification, therefore, is something I think we would all be well advised to do on a regular basis without waiting until we get sick. One of the reasons I suspect we don't take the cleansing process more seriously is that there is little conclusive and consistent data about how toxins and pollutants affect our health. How many of the studies that DO exist are funded by the companies who produce the chemicals in question? We know, for example, in the case of ALS and other neurological disorders, that a supposed connection exists between exposure to mercury and nerve damage. Yet some doctors who would be quick to point out that having amalgam fillings removed or undergoing chelation therapy to remove mercury from our bodies offers no consistently demonstrated potential for success in stemming or reversing neurological damage. Therefore, some people would choose to ignore the mercury levels in their bodies because removing it will not guarantee a reversal of their paralysis. This is simply another example of our endless yearning for the "magic pill." We always seem to be looking for the easy, convenient way out and the single cure that will clear the path to recovery.

The truth is that both disease and the human body are far more complex than that sort of thinking acknowledges. Many variables come together to cause an illness. We know, for example, that smoke, alcohol, and asbestos can all be contributing factors to cancer. We know that poor diet and lack of exercise can lead to obesity which, in turn, can lead to diabetes. In the case of an illness like ALS, however, where little clarity exists about its cause or cure, we can not afford to overlook any potential contributing factor. In my view, to dismiss or ignore the importance of mercury detoxification because it has not yet proven to be the "cure" for ALS is myopic, simplistic, and dangerous.

It is also important to remember that the human body is an amazingly complex and resilient organism with an inherent capability to heal itself when it is fueled and cared for properly. It is in our best interest, therefore, to learn as much as we can about how to protect it and ensure that its natural healing mechanisms are properly maintained. Removing and preventing the intrusion of toxins is key to ensuring that the body's natural capacities for self-healing can continue to operate optimally. For someone with ALS, this is imperative.

With this disease, I have to go to great lengths to minimize exposure to toxins. This includes some obvious measures, like avoiding fumes from auto exhausts, paints, pesticides, and cleaning chemicals—all of these things can trigger a crisis in my weakened state. I also read labels carefully to ensure that anything touching my body either inside or out contains only natural and, wherever possible, organic ingredients. This includes food, toiletry items, and household cleaning products.

I drink only highly filtered water from my own home. Processed foods, fast foods, and most cooked foods have been eliminated from my diet. I avoid exposure to microwaves and electro-magnetic waves wherever possible, by using distance and electronic diodes that interfere with the harmful effects of these waves.

In my efforts to remove built-up toxins from my body, I have had all my amalgam fillings removed, and employed both oral and intravenous chelation in order to reduce my exposure to mercury and other heavy metals. Oral use of a pill called DMSA and intravenous use of a substance known as EDTA have both helped me to chelate heavy metals, pesticides, and other toxins from my body. The most powerful method I discovered for removing heavy metals from the body is sound therapy. This astounding out-of-the-box technique for cleansing the body is worth looking into: passive listening through a pair of headphones to a series of tones for two hours a day, cut my mercury levels by more than 50 percent in only six weeks.

Another method I have used to remove toxins is mud packs. While this strategy is reportedly very powerful, I personally found it messy, time consuming, and unrewarding. Unlike sound therapy, it was difficult to consistently identify clear results from the hours spent mixing, wrapping, and rinsing mud. Perhaps if I lived nearer a hot springs instead of in the New Jersey suburbs it would have been different. An easier and more satisfying approach is the use of herbal patches on the reflexology points at the bottom of the feet. These patches, impregnated with herbs, can be purchased from doctors of Chinese medicine, some alternative practitioners, and through several sites on the Internet. Applied at bedtime, the pads become darkened by morning, suggesting they have absorbed toxins through the skin. I have used them with the intention of drawing toxins from my kidneys, liver, and colon. As with the mudpacks, however, it is difficult to obtain any scientific evidence of their effectiveness. The ABC news show, *20/20*, and several other institutions have conducted some small informal studies that found no evidence that these detox pads draw any identifiable toxins from the body. The only physical benefit I have derived from the use of the pads was increased relaxation of my legs, allowing for better sleep when I first began using them.

Probably the best overall method for cleansing and maintaining a healthy body is to feed it properly. Since we are constantly ingesting toxins through our food, air, and water, the purer the substances we put into our bodies, the fewer toxins we take in, and the greater chance we give our kidneys and liver to successfully perform the cleansing functions for which they were designed. Additionally, by eating properly we maintain an alkaline environment within our bodies. This is important because harmful bacteria and viruses thrive in acidic environments. By eating the right foods we balance our bodies for optimal energy, conditioning, and performance. Performance applies not only to athletic performance, but performance of our brains and immune systems. A nutrient-dense diet with minimal digestive effort helps us to maintain a system that is highly resistant to most causes of illness.

The problem with relying on diet alone to cleanse the body is that this ignores much of the toxic buildup accumulated during the years before starting a healthier practice. One of the most powerful approaches I have personally experienced for cleaning out stockpiled toxins was the lemonade diet, or Master Cleanser. This is an incredibly simple process that sounds far more challenging than it actually is, based on consuming nothing except a special blend of lemonade for a minimum of ten days. This lemonade consists of two tablespoons of freshly squeezed organic lemon juice, two tablespoons of pure organic maple syrup, and a tenth of a teaspoon of organic cayenne pepper in ten ounces of purified water. You can consume as much of this tasty mixture as you desire, but you must drink at least sixty ounces a day.

The process shuts down your digestive system, allowing your body to delegate more energy toward the removal of toxins, excess fat, mineral deposits, and hardened waste, and reestablishing an alkaline environment. Over the past decade specifically, the lemonade diet has been mislabeled and abused by some as a fad diet. Since it will shut down your digestive system after three or four days, it is not to be fooled with. There is an appropriate way to use it and an appropriate way to get back onto food when you are ready to complete your cleanse. If you plan to use this detoxing method, I strongly recommend that you first read a copy of *The Master Cleanser*, by Stanley Burroughs.

There are some incredible stories of turnarounds in cancer, kidney failure, and other serious health conditions just from using the Master Cleanser and other similar juice fasts. In my initial experience, I lived on this concoction for forty-nine consecutive days, consuming nothing else but water. Within the first year, I used the diet four more times, for a total of fifty-one additional days. When I began using the lemonade, I was at my weakest point in my battle with ALS, when no Western medical practitioner would have suggested fasting! But after completing one hundred days (not consecutively) on lemonade alone, diligently practicing affirmations for several months, and switching to a raw vegan diet, my weight began to increase and my energy level began to soar.

If you are in advanced stages of ALS and are considering giving lemonade a try, I strongly recommend that you find an experienced practitioner to assist you, as I did. In a weakened state, the intensity of this method of detoxification can create or reveal some challenging bumps in the road. Having someone by your side who has been down the path before is both helpful and comforting.

My most recent adventures with detoxification involved the use of a product called Miracle Mineral Supplement (MMS), which was developed by Jim Humble, based on years of research in Africa. After testing the supplement with tens of thousands of people, Humble has been able to show efficacy in reducing or eliminating the symptoms of a wide variety of ailments with MMS, including malaria, HIV, and numerous infections. The recipe consists of a simple solution of sodium chlorite, which, when mixed with a citric acid solution in proper proportions, converts to chlorine dioxide. When the chlorine dioxide enters the stomach, it triggers a massive oxygenation process. The increased oxygen molecules in the bloodstream destroy bacteria and viruses by attaching to, and breaking down, their cellular walls. They also carry off most pesticides, chemicals, and other pathogens for removal by the appropriate organs. The solution is purported to be effective in removing almost all known pathogens from the body. On the Internet, there is a world of information about the research findings, instructions for its use, and how to acquire MMS. Last but not least, it is dirt cheap. A year's supply can be acquired for about $30.00. Some fear that MMS is poisonous, but so are most medications when not used properly. My primary mechanism for assessing nutritional and toxicity issues during that time had been hair analysis, which indicates that MMS has been doing its job, but having done so much detoxifying with other methods, I cannot report feeling any significant physical effects from using MMS over the two years I used it.

I have intentionally omitted details on specific water filters, mud packs, cleaning solutions, toiletries, and other products. For such items, I have relied largely on the expertise of others. While I am happy to share the types of practices that are making a difference for me, I am reluctant to advise in areas that are outside my knowledge base. For some additional insights on how to deal with toxins and detoxification, I suggest a book called *Eric Is Winning*, by Eric Edney. While Mr. Edney's program differs from mine in some respects, he made positive strides in his battle with ALS (before dying of an unrelated heart attack at 85), and his thoughts may prove useful.

I am deeply concerned that our statistics in the United States on cancer, diabetes, heart disease, and obesity are among the highest on the planet. I find meaning in my battle with ALS by sharing what I have learned with others. Many in my sphere of influence are eating better, thinking more positively, cleansing more often, and generally taking better care of themselves as a result of what they have learned from my journey. If, through these pages, that influence and those results continue to expand, then my experiences with this illness will indeed have been worthwhile.

Optimal Nutrition

I am convinced that diet and nutrition are extremely important in fighting a chronic illness. This area of health management, however, is rife with controversy. As a result, relying on experts puts you at the mercy of each particular expert's bias, which can leave you dangerously at risk.

For example, during a visit to a clinic specializing in neuro-degenerative disorders, I was offered a lunch of tuna fish sandwiches and sugary fruit drinks. Tuna, as is well known, has one of the highest levels of mercury of any fish in the sea, and the health risks of processed or refined sugars are enormous. Sugar has been found to interfere with nutrient absorption, cause damage to the immune system and several vital organs, including the liver, pancreas and kidneys, and more. The ill effects of both mercury and sugar are well documented in numerous articles in medical journals and online.

In this same clinic, the nutritionist encouraged me to keep my weight up by ingesting high-caloric foods like Ensure and ice cream, both of which contain processed sugars. While I respect the professionals of this particular clinic and have found them to be helpful and supportive in many ways, their recommendations on nutrition appear to be frighteningly deficient, and downright dangerous.

One might wonder what would motivate well-intentioned and talented medical professionals to encourage the consumption of foods that include ingredients that are counterproductive, if not harmful, to the conditions of their patients. For me, the answer is quite simple. These professionals operate within a paradigm that assumes that their patients with ALS have no choice but to die. The only variables in their minds are how long it will take and how horribly they will suffer. Their focus, therefore, is not on what will actually make their patients better, but on what will keep them most comfortable as they waste away (and we all enjoy our sugary comfort foods). Their focus on nutrition, therefore, is to simply keep up caloric and protein intake in order to delay the "inevitable." The only hope in their thought process is that someday research will yield the magic bullet that will cure or control ALS. While hoping for this as well, I have no intention of waiting for it when there is so much more I can do to take care of myself.

One of the things that is clearly within my control is to eat properly. After ten or twelve years as a vegetarian before ALS struck, I thought that I was managing the nutritional aspects of my life quite well. My ALS diagnosis and the progressive deterioration of my body forced me to rethink what I knew about nutrition. After several years of experimenting, reading and yielding to the findings of my son's relentless research, my body's response to various dietary programs supplies the best evidence to support the wisdom of my current nutritional program for ALS. On this program, I have experienced more consistent and higher levels of general health and well-being, greater weight gain distributed throughout my body, and extraordinary increases in energy levels. It is not an easy program to transition to, but not terribly difficult to stay with once you have adapted to it.

The diet plan I follow is quite simple, consisting primarily of raw fruits and vegetables, with a heavy concentration on large quantities of a single fruit or vegetable at each meal. Organic sources of produce are used as much as possible. To learn more about this type of eating, I again recommend that you read *The 80/10/10 Diet*, by Douglas Graham, and *The Vegetarian Guide to Diet and Salad*, by Dr. Norman Walker. These two sources provide valuable information about what the body needs to function optimally. It is up to you, based on your results, to decide how much of their guidance you choose to follow.

An additional benefit of eating a highly nutritious diet is that it saves a lot of money on supplements. A number of other PALS (Persons with ALS) have claimed success in slowing or halting the progression of the disease through the use of various supplements like vitamin C, vitamin E, grape seed extract, beta carotene, selenium, Coenzyme Q10, B complex and others. While I have had little success with supplements (remember the days of 200 pills?)—I would not discourage other PALS from experimenting with them. It could be that, with enough detoxing, appropriate exercise, and positive energy work, a tailored protocol of supplements could be quite beneficial. Acquiring vitamins and minerals directly from whole raw fruit and vegetable sources has worked best for me. The only supplements I am currently using are MMS and an essential enzyme formula to enhance the absorption of nutrients from the foods I eat. I do keep an eye out for new supplements as well as pharmaceutical developments that might enhance the effects of my current regimen.

Exercise

Exercise and ALS are concepts that many people do not associate with one another. Doctors advise that mild cardiovascular exercise can be helpful, but that resistance training should be avoided by patients with ALS. Their thinking is based on the assumption that ALS is a one-way street of neural and muscular degeneration, and that resistance exercise will only hasten it. My personal experience has been that both mild cardiovascular and resistance exercise have helped to maintain my muscle tone and strength throughout the years. When either one has been eliminated from my regimen, atrophy has increased. It is also important to consider that I had exercised consistently, maintained a healthy weight, and eaten a relatively healthy diet before being diagnosed with ALS. Perhaps someone with a more sedentary pre-illness lifestyle might experience different results, based on the level of shock that the new implementation of such exercise might cause their system.

Similarly, I am fairly confident that the results of my exercise regimen would be less favorable without my current diet and other regular practices: intention and responsibility, detoxification, living in affirmation, and other forms of attracting healing energy. The current exercise routine includes a series of range-of-motion exercises, completed with assistance at the start of each day. Three or four afternoons a week, I lie across a rebounder while my aide straddles my hips and jumps up and down for several minutes to stimulate healthy cell activity. This is followed by bending and stretching of my arms and legs with assistance.

Occasionally, I do additional arm and leg exercises with the use of a Theraband suspended from a ladder straddled across the wheelchair. Once a helper positions my hand or foot in the sling created by the suspended Theraband (exercise rubber band), I can pull, push, or swing my arm or leg in different positions to exercise a variety of muscles. This activity enables me to achieve mild degrees of both cardiovascular and resistance exercise. Another form of cardiovascular activity that can be helpful is to employ a cough-assist machine or a spirometer to exercise the diaphragm and chest muscles. I know this sounds strange, but "Coughersize" is a novel but useful approach to cardiovascular exercise for someone with limited mobility.

In addition to all of this, I have found the use of a swing machine to be extremely helpful. This machine passively rocks the legs from side to side at various speeds, stimulating cellular activity as well as blood and lymph flow, and encouraging spinal alignment. Using this machine in the morning and before bedtime has increased circulation in my feet and legs, reduced swelling in my feet and ankles, and eliminated pain that previously kept me awake at night.

I would recommend acquiring input from exercise professionals to ensure that you are using the right exercises for your body and condition. Dr. Douglas Graham, author of *The 80/10/10 Diet,* has also provided valuable suggestions in building an exercise regimen, as well as managing diet. Assistance from professionals can save you time and energy of doing extensive research, and can help you avoid the dangers and time-sink of experimenting with the wrong exercises.

The Attraction of Healing Energy

Finally we come to the part of the formula that I consider most important. The generation and attraction of positive, healing energy creates a foundation that supports all of the other strategies discussed here. Maintaining a strong intention in the face of overwhelming challenges is impossible without constant affirmation of that intention. It is extraordinarily self-defeating to maintain a highly unusual diet, or to implement lifestyle changes to avoid toxic exposure, without a constant, positive focus on the benefits of such changes. Accepting responsibility for my mental activity, and diligently guiding that activity towards my goals of healing and happiness, have made a greater impact on my health and state of being than anything else. To put it another way, the Law of Attraction has worked well for me.

There are many ways to do this. Earlier, I described how the use of a gratitude list and affirmations has transformed the way I view my circumstances, and the "Healing Codes" energy healing meditations I work with to enhance both physical and spiritual functioning. This mental/emotional work has rapidly eliminated aches and pains from my joints, accelerated the healing of rashes, enhanced breathing, and dissipated long-held troublesome memories and beliefs resulting in a significant reduction of tensions and *dis-ease*, and a greater sense of *ease*.

I also experimented with a variety of healing medallions and energy-treatment devices and strategies, including working with a Journey practitioner, acupuncture, and healing stones (see glossary). While worthy of consideration, medallions and stones have not yielded clear enough results for me to offer a strong personal recommendation.

The Journey process is a strategy, based on NLP (see glossary), that I believe holds great promise. I have read Brandon Bay's *The Journey*, applied some of the concepts on my own, and am currently working with a practitioner on a regular basis. She guides and coaches me through the unearthing of emotions and visions related to memories that may have contributed to my current physical state. The theory is that by clearing these memories and releasing their hold on me, I can unleash the self-healing power of my mind and body.

Through this process, I have experienced a profound sense of contact with my inner being and a surfacing and dissipation of long-held beliefs and memories that I am convinced have contributed to my illness. While it is difficult to point to specific tangible results from this work, it seems to have contributed to increased energy and improvements in breathing. I am encouraged enough by the emotional impact of the experience to continue including this work as one of my strategies to promote healing.

Acupuncture is another method of using energy to promote healing that deserves serious consideration by anyone with illness. My initial experience with thin needles being placed in certain energy points on my body, described in Chapter 8, yielded little progress over a five-month period. Since that time, after considerable detoxing and dietary changes, acupuncture has become a staple of my treatment plan. Treatments keep my energy flow strong and help to prevent the recurrence of chronic pain from the deterioration of muscle tissue around the joints. My practitioner believes that building sufficient strength in energy flow may eventually translate into improved nerve and muscle activity. Indeed, the encouraging thing about my current acupuncture experience is that the increased energy levels I have traditionally gained from each session are now actually holding. Before I did my cleansing, spiritual, and psychological work, the increased energy I experienced after each treatment would dissipate before the next one. Eliminating toxins and improving my diet has created an opportunity for acupuncture to make a larger and longer-lasting contribution to my health. I am excited about the prospects.

Lastly, in the realm of technology, a vast array of electronic equipment holds promise for various types of physical healing. Beginning with the Rife Machine, a variety of frequency-detecting and -emitting devices exist that can both identify and resolve issues of toxicity and functioning within the body. While the logic behind the use of such instruments is quite sound, their effectiveness as part of a treatment program for ALS in general remains in question due to the lack of controlled studies to demonstrate their impact. Since such technology is not widely accepted in the U.S., it is also difficult to access good equipment and practitioners. Other than sound therapy, my personal experience with a number of these devices has been inconclusive.

> On Joe's 60th birthday, I wrote to him, 'The best thing I can say about you turning sixty is that you are doing so while totally confounding and confusing the bureaucrats who can't figure out why you have stayed on hospice care this long. May you continue to confound and confuse them for a long, long time!
>
> **GIL GORDON**
> LONGTIME FRIEND

But one piece of frequency-based equipment worth exploring is a device known as Ondamed. Ondamed frequency stimulation, combined with a patient's cognitive and non-cognitive participation, promotes relaxation, muscle re-education, and immune system health. In addition, Ondamed provides a wide array of diagnostic and prescription uses, such as relief from pain, stress, and inflammation. During my trips to Germany, I was frequently exposed to this technology, which is basically a hand-held machine that reads the frequency of a particular organ and if is not within normal range, sends the correct frequency into it to "re-train" it. These treatments removed or reduced pesticides and other toxins and even accelerated the healing of a viral infection. Ondamed has been available in the United States for several years now. If you can find a practitioner nearby, I believe it is definitely worth pursuing.

Although the danger in relying on technology can be similar to the lure of searching for the "magic pill," it is an exciting frontier to explore. Perhaps scientists will someday develop a pill or technology that can cure, or at least control, ALS. Until that day comes, investing too much time, money, or hope in equipment or pills would divert attention from responsibly managing one's spiritual, psychological, and nutritional health.

CHAPTER TWENTY-THREE:

Ongoing Challenges

Thoughts and events often occur in my life that rattle my convictions about healing and disrupt my focus on staying positive. It takes constant vigilance to ward off threats to my intentions. Among the offenders are: unexpected reminders of the emotionally painful aspects of my condition, like missing what I used to be able to do; physical discomforts, like pressure pains and rashes; and awkward and/or offensive reactions others have to my physical state. Any of these things can trigger an internal struggle that tests the strength of my beliefs and my ability to persevere.

I do miss many things: being able to answer the phone and door, being able to travel easily, standing and walking on my own two feet, jogging, skiing, tennis, golf—and simply being able to take care of myself. The list goes on and on. I miss being able to read books and magazines, open mail, pick fruit, and climb the stairs to visit what used to be my bedroom, where my wedding pictures hang; I have not been in that room for more than five years. I miss being able to get up and change a light bulb or fix a leaky faucet or a faulty switch. Yet, with all of this to think about, I rarely allow myself to dwell on what I miss. Doing so serves only to bring up sadness and negative emotions that make me feel weak and powerless.

Some might argue that it is important to grieve the loss, and I accept this point of view. However, full engagement in grieving can carry with it the assumption that the loss is permanent. I choose to surrender to the reality of the moment without relinquishing my beliefs in the possibilities of the future. Therefore, I grieve over, and surrender to, the loss of physical capabilities in this moment, while remaining grateful that I once owned those capabilities and am fully committed to reclaiming them.

So, when these thoughts emerge, I quickly shift my focus to what I *can* do, and all that I have to feel grateful for. What I can do is use my communication skills to get clear information from my family about the details of needed repairs in the rooms I can't visit. What I can do is call my former business acquaintance turned handy friend, Gil Gordon, and schedule a time for him to come and do the repairs. What I can do is be grateful that I have loving people in my life, like Gil, to do repairs that my body cannot currently handle.

• • •

One of the more disturbing, unexpected reminders of my current physical reality came in the summer of 2008. Diane and I were watching a movie called *The Diving Bell and the Butterfly*, a true account of the editor of a French magazine who, as the result of a stroke, had been left with a condition known as "locked-in syndrome." In this condition, the mind works perfectly well but the body has little or no movement, not unlike ALS. The only physical capability he retained was the movement of one eye.

I found the movie to be increasingly intense and uncomfortable to watch. After a while, I began to question, "Why am I watching this?" Tired, Diane was catching only glimpses of the film while lying prone on the couch, nodding in and out of consciousness. As a way to ease my discomfort with a story that struck too close to home, I glanced at her adoringly every few minutes. Watching her lie there in blissful somnolence—her reddish-blonde locks haphazardly strewn around her face—brought me a sense of peace. She was completely oblivious to my traumatic struggle to stay engaged with the movie while fighting back the tears and intense emotional identification with

> Of all the times Joe made me laugh out loud, this stands out in my mind: I was gluing together a broken drawer in his office desk, and the glue was particularly smelly. He was nearby and I said something about the odor, and said perhaps he should drive himself out of the room. "Yeah, who knows," he replied. "It might be toxic and might cause me to get some incurable motor neuron disease and I'd have to be confined to a wheelchair."
>
> **GIL GORDON**
> **GENEROUS FRIEND**
> **(WITH GOOD TOOLS)**

the protagonist. I longed to get up from my wheelchair, walk over to the couch, and lie down beside her. The urge was so strong that it nearly lifted me from the chair.

In my mind's eye, I see the fantasy unfold. I imagine myself gently taking her in my arms, being careful not to wake her. My heart pounds with excitement and warms with the flood of love that I still feel for this woman after more than thirty-six years of marriage. I clear the strands of hair from her face and plant a delicate kiss on her eye.

A loud angry scream from the movie screen shatters my fantasy, hurling my consciousness back into my mostly paralyzed body. "No, no, turn it back on! What are you doing?" the main character shouts in his mind at the hospital attendant who, without any attempt to determine the patient's desires, changes the TV channel from the soccer game he was wrapped up in to a children's cartoon show—and leaves the room. The completely paralyzed patient is left alone with the cartoons, lying helplessly in furious indignation. His left eye, the only part of his body that he can move, darts wildly around the room, searching frantically for help and/or justice as he silently screams his outrage.

As I watched and listened to him cry out at this incredibly insensitive and humiliating act, I writhed with the frustration and rage that I shared with him. The emotion stirred memories of numerous times in which, lacking sufficient air capacity to express my needs clearly and quickly, I had been subjected to the rash and inappropriate actions of would-be helpers. Yet, at least I was still blessed with the gift of speech. I can only imagine the intensity of frustration experienced by this man. It was incredibly difficult to wrench myself out of the moment, to separate from my identification with his negative emotions, and to focus on my gratitude for the advantages that my physical state afforded me over his. The experience taught me a

> All too often, we can find ourselves in frustrating situations that we have the ability to change. For some, however, the tendency to blame seduces us into giving up that ability and abdicating our responsibility. Instead, we need only to choose to resolve the tension, or remove ourselves entirely, to regain control of peace and happiness. Once again, we come back to the power of choice.
>
> **DAN WIONS**

very important lesson: when I find myself watching a movie or experiencing a situation that causes me extreme discomfort, I no longer sit there and ask myself, "Why am I watching this?" Instead, I turn off the movie or disengage from the situation.

• • •

A couple of years ago, I had a visit from a woman named Claire, who had Parkinson's disease. During the course of our conversation, as I was inquiring about how she'd been doing, she commented that she had good days and bad days. Then she said to me, "You know how it is." Her daughter, who is a good friend, had encouraged her to come and see me in the hope that I could somehow help her to develop a more consistently positive orientation in dealing with her disease. So my response to her was not, "Yes, I do know how it is." Instead, I told her, "Actually, I don't. You see, I don't allow bad days; I don't have time for them." I explained to her that, although I have bad moments, I choose to shift my perspective when they occur, rather than allow them to turn into bad days.

Not too long after that exchange, I had an experience that shook my conviction in the words that I had spoken to Claire that day. It reminded me how difficult it can be to stay focused on the positive and all that I have to be grateful for. Diane and I had turned in around 11 o'clock at night. A couple of hours later, as is typical, I was awakened by the urge to empty my bladder. In an effort to minimize the number of times that I am compelled to interrupt Diane's rest, I sleep with the urinal bottle positioned between my legs. This works reasonably well—except when the bottle gets too full, or when an errant pain or itching problem prevents me from dozing back off. On this particular night, there were a number of disturbances that combined to prevent my return to dreamland.

It began with my taking notice that the urine bottle was about to overflow, and I was not yet finished taking care of business. With great reluctance, I succumbed to the realization that I had no choice but to allow my own discomfort to disturb my beloved wife. As Diane stumbled around the bed in a half-sleep state to come to my aid, it became clearer to me that the issues that had disrupted my own sleep went far beyond the pressure in my bladder. I noticed that while my electric blanket was not operating sufficiently to keep my arms, chest, and torso warm, it was baking my entire backside. From the tips of my shoulders to the bottom of my buttocks, I was itching unbearably due to the perspiration. After dealing with the urine bottle, Diane rolled me on my side and dutifully applied some anti-itching remedies to quell the hyperactivity in my skin. With the itching on my back now under control, she returned me to my back and proceeded to adjust the various towels and pillows that my health aide had so carefully positioned before settling me in bed.

By the time we had completed this process, our return to sleep had already been delayed by some twenty minutes. When I do have to awaken Diane, my goal is to have every possible concern addressed at that time, to avoid having to wake her again. I pray, when these things happen, that the issues will be few. On this night, my prayers were not to be answered.

Exhausted from sleep deprivation, and the physical effort of moving me around in bed, Diane was desperate to return to sleep, but unfortunately, my various physical discomforts would not let that happen. I did my best to let go of the minor discomforts created by the repositioning of my torso. Addressing this issue, especially in her fatigued state, was something that I knew Diane did not have the strength to do. While annoying, it was something that I felt I could bear.

What I could not bear was the next explosion of itching that materialized on my scalp and face beneath the straps of the device that holds my breathing tube in my nose. Most nights, when these incidents occur, Diane quickly and lovingly scratches the itch or moves my arm or leg—whatever is necessary to make me comfortable and allow the quiet to return. But on this night the issues seemed endless. Reaching for the hairbrush to scratch my itching scalp, she almost broke it in half wrenching me free from my relentless uneasiness.

Praying for strength to tolerate the discomforts, my heart broke and guilt washed over me in response to her rare display of frustration. It is hard for me to see her in anguish. The drama moves me to question my intentions to heal. Am I acting out of courage and conviction in trying to bring about this unheard-of recovery? Or am I just being selfish, keeping her from moving on? Times like these make surrendering to the moment much more difficult to achieve. Sometimes the only remedy is anticipating a brighter tomorrow while trying to sleep.

• • •

As I have mentioned before, I am bothered when people react to me as if I were in bad shape emotionally. It must be difficult for those who care about me not to imagine what it would be like to be in my shoes. Often, they assume I am feeling as awful as they think they would if they were the one in the wheelchair. Pity is something I don't find comforting. In fact, I find it condescending. Compassion and appreciation of the situation work a lot better for me. Being treated as if I were the vibrant and functioning human being that I feel like inside works best of all.

It's an odd experience when someone tries to console me who has no clue what I am feeling or what I need. So many people approach me like they are walking on glass, trying to be delicate, trying to cheer me up. It can get irritating and even depressing. How do you tell someone who is well-intentioned and concerned that you don't need the pep talk, that the pep talk itself is presumptuous and demeaning? People don't realize that, in their efforts to console me, they are playing out their own fears and struggles in a "there but for the grace of God" scenario. I find pity unbearable. I don't have time for it.

If my life is to be shorter than expected, I have too much to do to sit around feeling sorry for myself, and absolutely no tolerance for such a waste of time. I'm a guy with a disease, but I am still *me*. I am not the disease or a victim of it. It is just something that I now have to cope with. I don't want people viewing me as, "the ALS patient, poor bastard." I want people viewing me as Joe, who happens to have ALS, but who is also a father, a husband, a management consultant, a friend, and many other things. The disease is part of who I am. It does not define me.

Joe coped with his illness with incredible grace and consideration of all those around him, rather than indulging in self-pity. During our times together, we discussed family, friends, caregivers, and the world around us, both seriously and in fun. He treated all those around him with incredible patience and compassion, even though there were probably times when he didn't feel it. He found the time and energy to write a book about his experiences and the people around him, something that most people in his condition wouldn't think of doing. And he was forever optimistic in his outlook.

DEBBIE LAMPF
LONGTIME FRIEND

Separating pity from the true love, concern, and desire to help that others express can also be difficult at times. People have offered and contributed so much. Hearing the words, and experiencing the reality that people need to help are two different things. As someone who has shaped his career around assisting others with their growth opportunities and obstacles, it has been a struggle and an incredible learning experience allowing myself to be taken care of. It's clear to me that people need to help as a way of showing they care. This is part of how they grieve and deal with their own sense of helplessness about my situation. It took me a while to realize that letting others help me do things that I could no longer do myself was a way of helping them.

CHAPTER TWENTY-FOUR:

Glimmers of Progress

And the Road Forward

In several places throughout this book, I have mentioned some of the positive changes that have resulted from my efforts to improve my health. I have talked about increases in my weight, breathing capacity and energy level, my greater ease in movement, and in the completion of tasks like brushing my teeth. Many issues of joint and muscle stiffness and pain have been resolved. It is a source of constant amazement to many of the medical personnel who visit me that I do not suffer from bed sores, given that I spend virtually all of my time on my back—either in my bed or reclining in my wheelchair. I have achieved a sense of peace and calm that enables me to face unexpected crises and setbacks with focus, deliberateness, and an ease that sometimes surprises even me.

I have emerged from the nightmare of belief that a horrible and untimely death was rapidly approaching. Several years after I was expected to be gone, I am still here and have enjoyed miraculous enhancements in my psychological, emotional, spiritual, and physical health. I've even started blogging at www.fromnightmarestomiracles.blogspot.com.

Yet, despite all of these improvements, I do experience occasional setbacks that test the strength of my belief in recovery. Over the past several years, while I have experienced some physical improvements, other things have deteriorated. For example, during the past year, my hand strength has improved—though every now and then, fatigue saps that strength. Although my breathing has been fairly stable and improving for two years, it has recently eroded to a mere ten percent of normal capacity, leaving me dependent on the Bi-PAP most of the time. During the brief periods when I go without it, I sometimes have to interrupt the activity (i.e. eating or brushing my teeth) several times for extra air before completing the task. Recently it has become harder to get through a meal without a morsel or two—or three—finding their way down my trachea. When this happens everyone gets to enjoy several minutes of coughing and gagging to clear it. At other times, I swallow my food and water with little difficulty. During the moments when things become more difficult, I find myself working harder on my gratitude list and affirmations to reinforce my resolve to heal.

Maintaining perspective seems crucial to the process of restoring my health. When I focus on day-to-day changes, the observations can severely challenge my perception of improved well-being. When I consider the past few years, however, my increased weight, energy, improved appearance, and ease of movement all reinforce my belief that I am winning the war against ALS.

Doctors may say that they have seen cases of ALS in which a patient goes through periods of improvement and decline several times in the course of the illness. On this basis, they might dismiss the role of my program in achieving the results I have cited. They might point to people like Stephen Hawking, who has survived with ALS for nearly fifty years without any specific, publicly documented treatment plan that I have been able to locate. What I have read about Stephen Hawking, however, is that he is a man with a strong personality and an intense lust for life and for his work. He once wrote that ALS has deprived him of little that he enjoys doing. Given that, one might argue that this is a man who lives in affirmation and that his affirmative orientation plays a significant role in his survival, though doctors say he has a rare variety of ALS.

I would love to see the results of a research study that assessed the level of the affirmative nature of ALS patients who survive the illness for ten years or more, compared to those who succumb quickly. Certainly there is much anecdotal evidence that a positive attitude and perseverance can contribute to an individual's success in overcoming health and other difficult issues. Many books have been written on this subject. Norman Cousins' book, *Anatomy of an Illness*, and other true stories cited in Chapter 18 are examples.

Some might dismiss the gains I cite here as slow progression or "burnout," a term some doctors use to describe the unexplained cessation of ALS progression. But I remember a night several years ago when I was carried to bed gasping for air, certain that I would not see the light of another day. I remember missing weddings and other events because I lacked the strength or the confidence to venture out of the house and participate. I remember frequently spending hours on the toilet in excruciating pain, trying to release my waste. Thanks to changes in diet, psychological orientation, the benefits of detoxification, exercise and spiritual healing, these occurrences are now nothing more than unpleasant memories.

Today, my body functions much more easily and with little discomfort. I am able to participate at weddings, graduation parties, and other celebratory events with confidence, and delight my friends and relatives with my wheelchair dancing. I go to movies, dine out, and even travel for overnight visits. I live with joy and the expectation of many tomorrows. My mental and physical states are very different than they were three or four years ago.

At this point in my adventure, I have grown certain that the key to full recovery lies in continued spiritual development. I am convinced that once I learn to completely unleash the natural self-healing powers of my body, complete health will be restored. It is my intention to pursue this goal until one of four things happens: one, I succeed; two, a true miracle drug emerges from the pharmaceutical world with the power to restore my mobility without serious side effects; three, I run out of time; or four, I get hit by the proverbial beer truck and we never get to know the true results of my efforts.

I have no crystal ball. I cannot know for certain what the future holds in store. It is my iron-clad conviction, however, that what I choose to believe has a primary and enormous impact on the part of my future that is within my control to create. So I choose to live my life as fully as I can, to do so in gratitude and affirmation of the many gifts and blessings that define my present, and with full intention of creating my desired future.

ALS is not a condition that I would have wished for, but it has launched me into an experience of extraordinary wonder, challenge, growth, and opportunity. It sometimes feels as if I have been whisked away into a different dimension, where gravity is stronger and the air is thinner. In this dimension, I find myself confronted by vast amounts of darkness, speckled with countless points of brilliant light, as if floating in space. The contrast presents me with soul-wrenching decisions to ponder. Do I succumb to the lure of the darkness? Do I give in to the oppressive weight of the intense gravity that renders my arms, legs, neck, and back all but totally immobile? Do I unplug the Bi-PAP that provides the only source of sufficient air pressure to keep my lungs functioning in this woefully thin atmosphere? It would be so much easier to just let it all go, to drift off into the darkness and let my soul move on to the next of its adventures through eternity.

On the other hand, there is the feeling of incompleteness in this current life; the sense that I have been torn away from the life I had known to fulfill some greater purpose. And what about all those countless points of brilliant light? What do they represent? Are they symbols of the hope for a cure, reflected in each breath laboriously drawn by every person struggling to survive another day with ALS? Are they opportunities flickering in the darkness and waiting to be explored, opportunities to expand humankind's capacity to deal with illness and other problems in more enlightened and productive ways? These are lofty thoughts. But, left with the choice of seeing myself as the victim or seeing myself as an unintentional astronaut poised to explore new frontiers...I choose the latter.

> These years provided challenges that gave me clarity on what life really means. To me, life is about love, living passionately, and learning to embrace our unique selves as we grow. It is valuing what we have and appreciating the precious individuals whom we choose to keep in our circle. It involves exploring how to simplify and discover what nurtures our inner peace and core being.
>
> **JULIE WIONS**

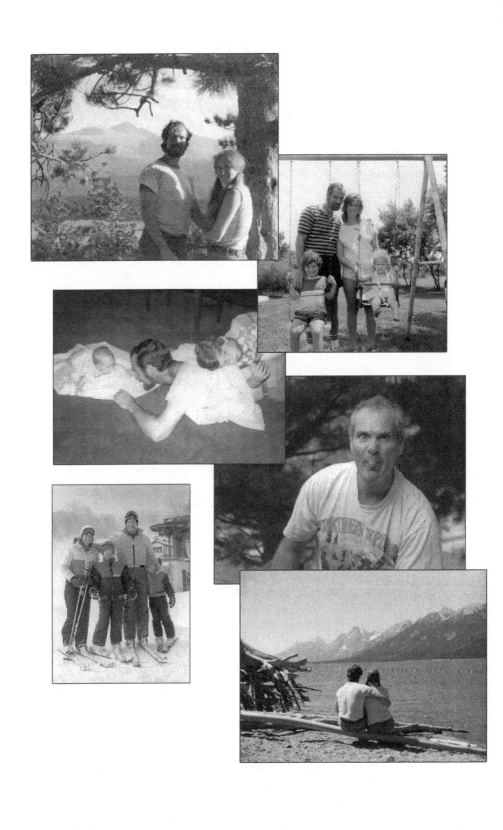

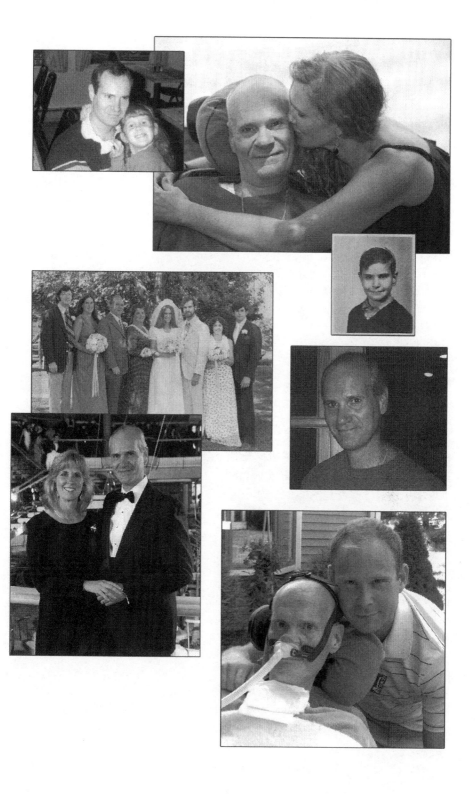

Afterword

After completing this manuscript, Joe continued to blog for several years about the continuing interplay of miraculous recoveries in one department, and the deterioration of others. He lost more hand and arm function, but then recovered it and also gained strength in his neck and shoulders. He celebrated his 60th birthday with a surprise party in the family's yard. Many friends, family, and former colleagues traveled to share in this celebration. Newspapers wrote about him as "Local Man Beating the Odds."

Yet, even as he began to turn the corner with health and mobility, ALS continued its creep in his throat. He would handle a three-hour coughing episode with cheeky responses like, "Are we there yet?" or "Let's do that again," connecting with his family and aides with his traditional humor. However, the deterioration of his epiglottis continued. He blamed himself for losing his focus and discipline with the hard work of healing, and re-instituted practices he had lost track of, such as meditation and mental trips to the gym. Eventually he decided to opt for a feeding tube surgery. When people began to have trouble understanding his "ALS accent," he acquired a device to help him speak (and change TV channels)!

He continued to write about all of

> Near the very end, when he needed to use an optical recognition computer to speak, Joe and I were outside and I was saying some negative things about Obama. After I was finished, I said to him "It's too bad you can't speak Joe, because now you can never defend him to me anymore." Suddenly the device voice came back with "Fuck you, Asshole!" I couldn't stop laughing.
>
> **HOWARD GUTTMAN**
> COLLEAGUE AND FRIEND

these experiences in his blog, ranting about "medical myopia"—the pain of being ignored when you can't verbally interact with people at their level—and sharing new treatment options with the ALS community. He worked with other pioneers in the HALS (Healers of ALS) community, re-evaluating his processes and exploring dietary and psychological changes based on the success of others.

Adjustments to the new feeding tube caused Joe to lose weight and strength, and writing became more difficult. He adapted to the new level with positivity, however, and committed to writing a blog post each month. He wrote, "Hopefully all of this will change soon. Until it does, I will try to get out a post at least once a month." In retrospect, the word, "try" seems especially poignant.

Joe wrote in his last blog post:

```
"Recently, while trying to comfort another HALS
member, I mentioned that I rarely allow myself
more than a few moments in a depressed state. In
the past few months, this belief has been
challenged several times. Just last week, a trip
to the emergency room for dehydration coming from
some ill-considered premature changes to my diet,
shook my convictions. An ill-conceived
prescription (something that I don't often take)
worsened my condition, causing me to suffer for
days with severe stomach pain. Throughout this
ordeal, I have struggled to fend off thoughts of
losing my battle with ALS, and fighting to refocus
on my intention, affirmations, and healing
practices. It has been incredibly difficult.
Fortunately, as the pain has eased, so has the
struggle. I finally feel like I am getting back on
track.

Moral of this story: it is easier to follow your
intention when you are feeling well, but without
one, you may become totally lost."
```

Joe passed away in his sleep on July 27th, 2011. Dan wrote, "Over the past 11 years, I have seen my Dad appear seconds away from death more times than I would like to count. I have seen his skin turn gray, his eyes glaze over, and his breathing stop. In the past, due to fainting spells brought on by treatments or a lack of oxygen, Mom, Julie or I have revived him from this state. So when my mom came into my room at 7:45am, and said, 'I think Daddy died,' I went into productive mode. I raced downstairs, I examined his body...I saw the same glazed eyes and gray skin. The breathing machine was still pumping air into his lungs. It was almost as if I could just shake him and snap him out of it. But his pulse was gone. I felt cheated. We had made it so far, only to give up now. His intent was still strong. I mean, he was terrified, more than most people knew, but he was continuing to evolve and heal in so many ways, and he still wanted to live. The whole thing was so surreal."

Joe's funeral was packed by the incredible community that had supported and loved him for so long. After living with such an intense version of "normal" for so long, it took some time to re-adjust. The week after Joe died, Dan observed a single wild turkey coming and sitting under the bay window, where, day after day, Joe had enjoyed watching his "wildlife special" unfold in the back yard. "From what I understand," wrote Dan, "turkeys travel in flocks. But this one was all alone, and it came every day, sometimes accompanied by a pair of doves."

Julie, who had moved back home to help support her family, finally pursued her dream to move to California and start her artistic career. She wrote, "A month before Dad died, as the health aid was assisting and cleaning him, I lay on the bed facing him. In his eyes, I saw so much depth—love, fear, pain, loss, and acceptance. There was nothing I could do to take his pain away. I whispered to him how much I loved him, and he whispered right back 'I love you, Julie.' His words became slurred. But the day I drove across the country, I took his voice with me."

> The morning before I left for California, Mom came into my room and called me her "little pioneer." She told me how much I reminded her of Dad when he was my age, taking the same brave adventures. So, as I got in my car and drove off in search of my independence, I thought of Dad and how privileged I felt to follow in his footsteps and carry a part of him with me. Recently looking through some old albums, I noticed a picture that he took at Bryce Canyon in his early 20's during his travels. I didn't discover until after that I had stood in the same spot and had taken the exact same picture 35 years later.
>
> **JULIE WIONS**

That fall, Dan wrote in a blog post about the family, "Summer is over. It's now autumn, which means students, rehearsals, and performances. It's time to give more hugs, smile at strangers, and make beautiful music. It's time to be present, laugh every chance I get, take a step off the merry-go-round, and just keep walking."

On the one-year anniversary of Joe's passing, Julie was reflecting on her father and decided to spend the day celebrating his life. She awoke to an extraordinary experience that felt like a warm sign from beyond.

"My father loved birds. Every morning he'd sit in his wheelchair and meditate by the window observing these beautiful creatures. Hummingbirds were among his favorite, and anytime I see one I feel a connection to him. These mystical birds generally symbolize vitality, joy, renewal, sincerity, peace, as well as persistence, agility, playfulness, loyalty, and affection—all traits that remind me of my father. On the one-year anniversary of his passing, I woke up to discover a hummingbird had flown into the house and could not find his way out. Eventually, the poor thing tired out, and perched himself on the door ledge to regain his energy. When I reached up, the little hummingbird allowed me to hold him. I walked outside to set him free, but the bird stayed resting in my hand for a while. So for a few minutes before flying onto his next adventure, I got to treasure this gift, a beautiful reflection of my father's intense journey."

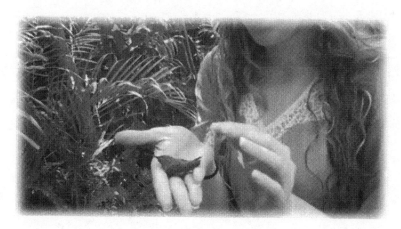

Joe's Legacy

After his diagnosis, Joe dedicated his life to the belief that ALS can be overcome. Joe's family worked alongside him, and continue to work to move this dream forward for others affected by the disease.

SerenAIDe

Throughout the time of Joe's illness, Diane Wions' choir students at J.P. Stevens High School, in Edison NJ, produced a benefit concert that featured teachers, other students, community members, and alumni of the school. Proceeds from the concert went toward ALS research and helped the Wions family, as well as others fighting ALS.

This concert has become an annual event that brings together the community, builds confidence in kids, and creates beautiful and moving musical experiences. Footage is available through a quick Google or YouTube search of "SerenAIDe JP Stevens." To date, they have raised more than $75,000 for ALS research and support for families affected by the disease.

See www.facebook.com/SerenAIDe.

> SerenAIDe has become so much more than a benefit concert. It is about the community. It has united the township of Edison as a family. It has become about strength, hope, never giving up, and about pursuing your dreams— themes we have had throughout the years. It has sent such a powerful message to everyone that we have each other. It has impacted generations and put things into perspective. It reminds everyone that there are people willing to stand by you no matter what. I think that is one of the most important things in life.
>
> **KIRK GERITANO**

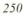

Julie Wions

Now a Los Angeles-based model and actress (www.juliewions.com), Julie displays her moving and insightful original artwork and photography on her website, www.creationsbyjulie.net. A portion of all profits from your purchase of her products is donated to the ALS Association, to support the fight against Lou Gehrig's Disease. Like her father, Julie is passionate about helping others in her community. She works part time as a residential technician for victims of abuse, trauma, mental illness and addiction, and volunteers for the homeless on her time off.

Dan Wions

Dan continues to work as a professional musician, playing French horn in orchestras all over the world. Dan also refers musicians for projects and events through his company, Live Music Consulting. Meet Dan on his website, www.livemusicconsulting.com.

Dan wrote a piano piece, entitled *From Nightmares to Miracles,* which was the working title of this book. The song premiered at the last SerenAIDe concert before Joe's death, on May 27th, 2011. You can see this performance on youtube at tinyurl.com/dan4joe. And if you listen closely, you can hear the periodic beeping of Joe's Bi-PAP machine in the front row.

You can get *From Nightmares to Miracles* on iTunes.

> Growing up, people would tell me how much I sounded like my Dad more and more each year, whether because of a corny joke I'd let slip, or just the sound of my voice alone. This would usually draw a groan from me and laughter from everyone else. Today, I could not be more proud to remind people of this wonderful man.
>
> **DAN WIONS**

From Nightmares to Miracles

Joe's blog contains many more links, suggestions, stories…and comments by more inspiring people! You can read more of his writing and add your thoughts at www.fromnightmarestomiracles.blogspot.com.

> Inspiring… Nothing short of inspiring!
>
> **KIM**
> **BLOG COMMENT**

All of the information below can be accessed at
www.MoreTimetoLove.com.

Acknowledgments

Words that adequately express the depth of my gratitude simply don't seem to exist. I live in constant awe of the blessings of my family and friends, and from an army of allies, supporters, and well-wishers. These people have done everything from helping to keep my family financially stable to assisting me with personal care in the bathroom. I cannot read this list without getting emotional. Even more awesome is the fact that the list is incomplete. My full-hearted gratitude goes to everyone who contributed—those mentioned here, and those not mentioned.

Luz Acosta • Elaine and Howard Albert • Mitch and Gail Albert • Wendy Barnes • Richie Bencivenga • Bess Berg • David and Jann Berg • Carol Bocchino • Ida Breitbart • Jim and Joanne Bunce • Dona Lee Calabrese • Susan Carson • Harvey Cavayero • Morris and Rita Cavayero • Ronnie and Steve Charme • CKS Hebrew School • Michaele and Tom Divito • David and Lisa Dvorin • Carol Dyer • Judi and Ed Edelson • Pete Elder • Rabbi Susan Falk • Bob and Peggy Fass • Jo Ann Ferraro • Janis Fisher • Walt and Zoe Fuller • Gisele Garcia • Gil Gordon • Scott Gordon • June Halper • Howard and Jackie Guttman • Roger Holdredge • Joe and Paula Horowitz • Gail Houseman • Janet James • Nancy and Mitch Javelin • Li and Hong Jin and Nicholas Jin • Charlotte Johnson • Carol and Frank Jones • J.P. Stevens High School Choir and COPA • Fred and Randi Katzman • Mary Kelly • Lisa Kent • Dr. Wolf-Dieter Kessler • Jennifer Klapper • Nick Klevans • Tim and Leslie Kowalski • Bonnie Kramer • Wendy Krasner • Ellen Kratka • Marty Kurtz • Debbie Lampf • Lisa Larson • Sue Lawton • Valerie Lemme • Judi Lewis • Don Linford and family • Natalie London • Joel and Jane Lubin • Alan Marcus • Rabbi Shana Margolin • Dr. Leo McCluskey • Dan and Sue Mitchell • Joan Montanari • John Moyle • Judi and Don Nickelson • Larry and Arlene Nieman • Shelley Nord • Klaus Oebel • Tamara Olson • Jim Ohls •

Meryl Orlando • Dan Parillo • Stan and Tobie Parnett • Raul, Lee and
Raymond Pedraja • Hongbo Qi and Ed Yang • Thom Radice • Phyllis
and Phil Remolador • Bobbie and Marty Resnick • Mirah Riben •
George Rieger • Marc and Harlene Rosenberg • Sheryl and Richard
Rosenberg • Matt Rosenthal • Jeff and Paula Ross • Eileen and Mike
Rothstein • Ralph Russo • Anton and Gerda Samuels • Hope and Lee
Schraeter • Eileen Schreibman • Josh Schreibman • Susan Schwartz •
Bruce and Anna Sherling • Eric and Leslie Sherling • Michael and
Dawn Sherling • Lloyd Smith • Steve Smotrich • Ling, Jake, and Kevin
Song • John and Sue Stagg • Rabbi Michael Tayvah • Debbie Tesser •
Bruce and Katie Vatter • Mary Wasserman • Barbara Weber and Jim
Kenny • Joan and Joel Weisblatt • Tom Woloshyn • David Wions •
Kristina Wise • Lenny and Mona Witman • Lewis and Karen
Wolkofsky • Maureen Woods • Dr. Fen Xie • Jess and Rick Zendt •
Heidi Zorde

A special note of thanks to those who read and critiqued my first
draft. Their feedback helped crystalize the original framework, and
shape and strengthen the focus for this book. This included my cousins,
Joe and Paula Horowitz; my friends, Jim Bunce, Peter Tobia, Dale
Corey, Howard Guttman, Gisele Garcia, and Jo Ann Ferraro; my wife,
Diane; my son, Dan: and my daughter, Julie. Last, but not least I want
to acknowledge my friend, Joan Montanari, whose on-going assistance
with typing, editing, and added perspective have enhanced the quality
of this writing and speeded its development.

On Joe's behalf, Dan and Julie would like to add their gratitude to
Kristen Caven and Louise Hart at Uplift Press for all of their efforts to
get this book into your hands. Also thanks to Juliana Pereira and Pete
Larson.

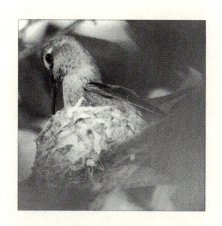

Appendices

Resources for People with ALS

The purpose of this section is to share my thoughts on some pragmatic issues with which people are faced once they are given the diagnosis of ALS. I want to emphasize that these are my thoughts, based on my personal experience, beliefs, and biases. My hope is that by sharing my learning and conclusions I will save others facing ALS some critical time in finding the resources they need.

Choosing a doctor:

Your choice of doctor depends on the choice you make about how to deal with ALS. If you choose to follow conventional treatment, find the best and most experienced motor-neuron specialist within your geographical reach. Make sure that your neurologist's office is affiliated with a clinic that offers you one-stop shopping for services. You will want to have access to occupational therapists, physical therapists, throat specialists, respiratory therapists, nutritionists, and social workers all in one place. Another consideration is the doctor's affiliation with support organizations like ALSA (ALS Association) and MDA (Muscular Dystrophy Association). These organizations can provide access to information on a wide variety of resources, including home-modification experts, durable medical equipment resources, financial aid programs, and more.

If you choose a more adventurous path that includes the use of alternative medical resources, the recommendation above still stands— but with some additional considerations. While many traditionally trained physicians pay lip service to the idea of integrating alternative practices with traditional medicine, I have met few who were actually willing to invest time and energy into learning enough to support my efforts.

The more open, willing, and involved your neurologist is in helping you integrate these two worlds of medical practice, the faster your progress will be in finding a formula that works for you. I encourage you to ask your prospective choice of physician what his or her experience has been in integrating traditional and alternative practice.

Advice on home modifications and repairs:

Through your doctor's clinic or organizations like ALSA and MDA, you can find recommendations for people who specialize in home modification to prepare for living with declining physical abilities. These people generally work for a consulting fee. They will come to your home, assess your needs, and leave you with recommendations on everything from installing grab bars and ramps to widening doorways and acquiring facilitative equipment.

Another resource worth pursuing is a good care manager. These individuals can either advise you on home modifications or find you someone who can, as well as help you locate other resources like home health aides. These people also generally work on an hourly-fee basis. If you find one early in the game, he or she can save you a tremendous amount of time and energy, and can become a valuable long-term ally in acquiring resources, particularly if your disease progresses in a way that makes it more difficult for you to do the research on your own.

Where to get durable medical equipment:

Costs for durable medical equipment can vary widely. You can spend as little as ten or twelve dollars for a grab bar, fifty to a hundred dollars for an adaptive toilet seat, several hundred dollars for a portable ramp, or twenty-five thousand dollars for a power wheelchair. While most of this equipment is readily available through medical supply stores and some pharmacies, most people do not have the assets to pay the formidable expenses for durable medical equipment that can be needed.

Through an affiliation of the doctor's neurology clinic with support organizations like ALSA and MDA, patients may have access to "loaner closets." Local medical equipment supply businesses may have a supply of donated, used equipment that they will provide free of charge to patients in need. In some cases, if equipment is needed and not available in loaner closet supplies, the ALSA or MDA chapter will purchase and provide it on loan to the patient. The only requirement is that the equipment be returned when it is no longer needed.

Creating a support network:

As you might surmise from my book, there is nothing more important than a good support network. The good news is, it is never too late to build one. I have met some unfortunate souls with ALS who believe that there are few people out there who stand ready to provide help. They believe that since they have not devoted effort in their pre-ALS lives to supporting others, they have no one to call on in their time of need. Certainly those who have helped others are more likely to receive support in return. But if you are like me, the hardest part about dealing with your support network will be learning how to accept the support.

It is important to understand, however, that getting the support you need is not a matter of calling in some social debt. People by nature are generally compelled to help when they see someone in need, and may see it as an opportunity to do something meaningful. There are individuals and organizations all around you who are ready and willing to do so the moment they know what is needed. Friends and family are usually the first to step up. Following close behind are members of religious congregations. Then there are organizations whose reason for existing is largely to provide support and resources. I have already cited some of the help available through doctors' clinics and organizations such as ALSA and MDA. There may also be local programs available in your community. Your municipal government may provide programs such as transportation for disabled residents and free handyman services. There are also grant programs available to help pay for things like home health care, such as the Care for Life

Program, which provides a one-time grant for respite care to relieve family caregivers.

As you draw people and organizations into your support network, your orientation toward your illness becomes increasingly important in sustaining relationships. The more you see yourself as a victim, the harder it is for people to continue to be there for you.

Think about someone in your life who has fallen on hard times and has reacted to it by wallowing in misery, depression, and self-pity. What was it like to be around them? As much as people want to help, by projecting pain you make it more difficult for them to do so. Keep in mind that you are a person with an illness. *You are not the illness.* The extent to which you continue to live your life and adapt to your changing circumstances will inspire and motivate others to want to help.

It is also important to recognize that, in doing so, you are not taking advantage of them. On the contrary, you are opening possibilities for them to do good as they ease your burden. There is no greater gift in life than to empower people to make contributions that make them feel good. As you are receiving, you are also giving. Accepting the gift of support is not a one-way street. And remember, it is never too late to build and contribute to a support network.

There are many online support networks for those with ALS. They can't replace real people in your life. Sadly, most real people don't know what you are going through like your online friends. Some of my go-tos:

- alsa.org - find your local chapter at alsa.org/community
- ericiswinning.com
- healingwithdrcraig.com

Home health aides:

Finding, training, and keeping a good home health aide can be far more of an adventure than anyone in need would want it to be. The hourly cost of a health aide can range from $12 to $30. Live-in rates can range from $100 to $250 per day. Rates vary with the degree of training and experience, whether you go private or through an agency, and on the degree of risk you are willing to tolerate.

Agencies are usually more expensive because, like any business, they have overhead expenses. While they save you the effort of screening and ensuring appropriate credentials, there is no guarantee of quality. On the other hand, when you go private, you have to be careful to avoid potential legal and security issues. Most home health aides come from other countries and are trying to establish themselves financially in the U.S. If the aide is not yet a citizen and comes to you through an agency, you can rest assured that they have already acquired a green card and they are probably bonded. When you hire privately, this is not always the case. The last thing you need, in addition to managing a serious illness, is finding yourself being complicit in aiding and abetting an illegal alien or finding yourself in a situation where you are being mistreated, abused, or robbed by a person who is supposed to be caring for you. So, make sure your aide has a green card or citizenship, and check out experience and references.

Among the most important qualities to look for in a home health aide are communication skills. Since most are foreign born, even those who were brought up speaking English may have accents and cultural nuances to the language that can make arriving at mutual understanding an unwanted adventure. This is an adventure that you would clearly prefer to avoid, especially when you need to be moved out of a position that is causing you pain, and you are too short of breath to speak louder than a whisper.

A second quality that I have found to be critical is that the health aide is doing that job because he or she loves the work. Many immigrants take on live-in health aide work because it is one of the best-paying jobs they can find upon arrival in this country. It only requires about twelve weeks of training to acquire a CHHA (Certified Home Health Aide) certificate, and live-in work eliminates the need for personal transportation. Since many people doing this job cannot afford cars, it is a perfect fit. All of this is fine as long as the individual also enjoys the work.

Whenever a new aide begins working for me, I always take time to learn something about his or her background and interests. Among the things I want to know are how long they have been doing health aide work, how they got into it, and what they most like about it. During one changing of the guard, a new aide responded to my inquiry about how he liked the work with, "It's better than nothing." I knew immediately that this meant trouble, but out of concern that I would not be able to replace him immediately, I tried to ignore my instincts and give him a chance. In less than 24 hours, I had to ask him to leave. Rather than paying attention to the training process, he did nothing but complain about the difficulty of the job, creating a great deal of stress and wasting my time and effort to train him. The most effective aides I have had came with a history of experience in, and attraction to, health care. These people are almost always extremely attentive and easy to train.

In addition to communication abilities and affinity for the work, there are several other criteria I have found useful. Always think through, in advance, the criteria you are using to evaluate a potential aide. Keep these criteria firmly in mind if you have the chance to interview a prospective aide in advance of the hire. If you don't have the opportunity to interview the aide yourself, you should provide a list of your criteria to your care manager or the agency you are working with. Following is the list I have shared with my care manager. Whenever the time comes to search for a new aide, this list guides our conversations in evaluating each candidate. I hope you find it useful.

Health Aide Selection Criteria

Communicates Effectively

Demonstrates ability and willingness to listen and assert self to ensure mutual understanding of needed support and responsibilities. Takes the extra step to ensure that language and cultural differences do not prevent understanding.

Enjoys the Work

Exhibits a sense of compassion, purpose and enthusiasm. Explains the choice of home health care over other types of work. Cares about people and takes pride in doing even the smallest tasks well and thoroughly. Takes initiative to get things done and make things better.

Time Management

Is able to accomplish a variety of tasks within a specified time frame. Is punctual when asked to begin or complete a task.

Attentiveness and Focus

Notices subtle signs that assistance may be needed. Does not leave client alone without ensuring all needs are met. Makes the client a priority and does not allow distractions (e.g., TV and phone calls) to get in the way.

Cleanliness

Pays attention to the condition of the home and does what is needed to keep it clean. Does not have to be asked, for example, to pick up litter but does so instinctively. Keeps all work and personal areas clean and organized. Uses appropriate measures to keep client safe from contamination and exposure to germs.

Adaptability and Willingness to Learn

Is willing and able to follow clear instructions without argument or defensiveness. Takes on new or usual tasks without complaint or attitude.

Financial help:

When I was about 40 years old, I had looked into long-term-care insurance. Being in fairly good health at the time, I decided I could risk a few more years before shelling out $3,000 a year for something I might never need. In retrospect, this was obviously not one of my better decisions. If you are still in a position to acquire such insurance, please learn from my mistake. If you were smarter than I was, and purchased a good long-term care policy *before* being diagnosed with a serious illness, your financial worries should be far less. If you have been diagnosed with ALS and plan on going with conventional treatment, your prescription plan and medical insurance should take care of many of your needs.

The biggest expenses you will incur in living with ALS are home modifications, durable medical equipment, home health aides, and alternative treatments. Long-term care insurance will take care of the health aide issue if you have enough coverage. Your local chapter of ALSA or MDA, as explained above, can probably take care of most of your durable medical equipment needs. What is not provided by their loaner closets may be covered by your medical insurance.

Home modifications, or a move into a more accessible living environment, also require assets or financial support. In extreme situations, where assets are not available, you may have to consider Medicaid and a nursing home, or an assisted living facility. Unfortunately, Medicaid only becomes available once you are down to your last couple of thousand dollars in assets. It may not be true across the country, but I do know that in some states, once you are Medicaid-eligible, you can enter a nursing home in return for your Social Security check.

For most alternative treatments, you will have to rely on your own assets or the generosity of others. Some medical plans will cover acupuncture and some forms of spiritual/energy treatment when performed by a medical professional. A portion of the cost for my initial experience with "Journey work," for example, was covered by my insurance company because it was performed by a psychiatrist. The only other treatments I have described in this book, for which I was able to acquire reimbursement through my medical insurance, were neuro-biofeedback and sound therapy. However, the insurance company gave me a great deal of difficulty and eventually cut off reimbursement at a fraction of my cost.

You have nothing to worry about if you are independently wealthy. But, if you are not, there is still no reason to panic. As I said earlier, people are only too willing to help once they recognize a need.

In order for them to do so, the person in need must be visible to those who stand ready to assist.

So how do you become visible? You begin by considering all of the people and organizations with whom you are connected. Friends and family are often eager to help in whatever way they can. All they need to know is how. Contact any local civic groups or religious organizations, like Knights of Columbus, Rotary Club, Jaycees, Jewish Family Services, or Lions Club that you may belong to or know of, as well as the clergy or other key representatives at your place of worship. You can also contact local and state agencies like County Social Services, Community Visiting Nurses Association, and your township or city government. Let them know your situation and what you can use in the way of assistance. Ask them to keep you informed of any financial aid resources of which they may be aware and for which you might be eligible. If you have been active in such organizations, chances are there is little else you will have to do before support starts to come your way.

Books:

The next Appendix contains a list of books and videos that I have found helpful. They include information on diet, cleansing and detoxification, the practice of affirmations, meditation, color therapy, Vitaflex, essential oils, the Law of Attraction, the Journey, and other spiritual healing practices. There are also several works about the experiences of others with ALS. I hope you find them to be as helpful as I have.

APPENDIX 2:

Bibliography

Albom, Mitch. *Tuesdays with Morrie: an Old Man, a
    Young Man, and Life's Greatest Lesson.* New York:
    Broadway, 2007.

Arntz, William, Betsy Chasse, and Mark Vicente. *What the
    Bleep Do We Know!?: Discovering the Endless
    Possibilities for Altering Your Everyday Reality.*
    Deerfield Beach, FL: Health Communications,
    2007.

Bays, Brandon. *The Journey: a Practical Guide to Healing
    Your Life and Setting Yourself Free.* New York:
    Atria Paperback, 2008.

Bays, Brandon. *The Journey: an Extraordinary Guide for
    Healing Your Life and Setting Yourself Free.*
    London: Harper Element, 2003.

Burroughs, Stanley. *Healing for the Age of Enlightenment:
    Balanced Nutrition, Vita Flex, Color Therapy.*
    Reno, NV: Burroughs, 1993.

Burroughs, Stanley. *The Master Cleanser: with Special Needs and Problems*. Auburn, CA: Bourroughs, 1993.

Byrne, Rhonda. *The Secret*. New York: Atria, 2006.

Edney, Eric. *Eric Is Winning!!: Beating a Terminal Illness with Nutrition, Avoiding Toxins and Common Sense*. Xlibris, 2004.

Graham, Douglas N. *The 80/10/10 Diet: Balancing Your Health, Your Weight, and Your Life One Luscious Bite at a Time*. Key Largo, FL: FoodnSport, 2006.

Hay, Louise L. *You Can Heal Your Life*. Carlsbad, CA: Hay House, 2004.

Kabat-Zinn, Jon. *Full Catastrophe Living: Using the Wisdom of Your Body and Mind to Face Stress, Pain, and Illness*. New York: Delta Trade Paperbacks, 1990.

Kabat-Zinn, Jon. *Wherever You Go, There You Are: Mindfulness Meditation in Everyday Life*. New York, NY: Hyperion, 2005.

Martin, Joe, and Ross Yockey. *On Any Given Day*. Winston-Salem, NC: John F. Blair, 2000.

Nieto, Augie, and T. R. Pearson. *Augie's Quest: One Man's Journey from Success to Significance*. New York: Bloomsbury, 2007.

Perlmutter, David, and Carol Colman. *The Better Brain Book: the Best Tools for Improving Memory and Sharpness and for Preventing Aging of the Brain.* New York: Riverhead, 2005.

Tolle, Eckhart. *A New Earth: Awakening to Your Life's Purpose.* New York: Plume Book, 2005.

Tolle, Eckhart. *The Power of Now: a Guide to Spiritual Enlightenment.* Vancouver, B.C.: Namaste Pub., 2004.

Wakefield, Darcy. *I Remember Running: the Year I Got Everything I Ever Wanted--and ALS.* New York: Marlowe, 2006.

Walker, Norman Wardhaugh. *The Vegetarian Guide to Diet & Salad: for Use in Connection with Vegetable and Fruit Juices.* Prescott, AZ: Norwalk, 1995.

Woloshyn, Tom. *The Complete Master Cleanse: a Step-by-Step Guide to Maximizing the Benefits of the Lemonade Diet.* Berkeley, CA: Ulysses, 2007.

Glossary

Acupuncture   A key component of traditional Chinese medicine involving thin needles inserted into the body at designated points along the body's energy meridians.

Affirmations   Positive statements that describe a desired situation can be repeated until they become "facts" to the subconscious mind. This process engages the mechanics of the subconscious, which will then work to make the positive statement come true.

Babinski Reflex   This reflex occurs after the sole of the foot has been firmly stroked. The big toe then moves upward or toward the top surface of the foot. The other toes fan out. This reflex is normal in children up to 2 years old. It disappears as the child gets older. When the Babinski reflex is present in a child older than 2 years or in an adult, it is often a sign of a brain or nervous system disorder.

Bi-PAP Machine   A non-invasive form of therapy for those who require breathing assistance. BiPAP stands for Bilevel Positive Airway Pressure, and is very similar in function and design to a CPAP machine (Continuous Positive Airway Pressure). BiPAP provides two different strengths of continuous positive airway pressure, whereas CPAP only has one strength setting.

Bodywork   A "hands on" process where the practitioner works with a patient to release chronic tension and rigidity in the body. All types of bodywork, from massage to chiropractic to rolfing, result in a more improved posture, greater flexibility and ease, and less physical discomfort.

BuNaoGao This Chinese herb formula, also known as 'BNG', is a purported to be helpful in the treatment of ALS and other degenerative conditions.

Brain Patterns Neurological deterioration can be measured with certain techniques using an MRI machine. A known set of functional cerebral abnormalities are monitored in ALS patients.

Chelation An oral or intravenous treatment that removes metals from tissues. The word *chelate* comes from the Greek root chele, which means "to claw." EDTA has a claw like molecular structure that binds to heavy metals and other toxins.

Color Therapy A Frequency Treatment involving the use of different colors (light frequencies) to treat the body. *The Master Cleanse*, by Stanley Burroughs, is a published chapter from a larger work entitled "Healing for the Age of Enlightenment," which includes a detailed chapter on Color Therapy. Color Therapy is also used in conjunction with some Frequency Treatments.

DMSA Dimercaptosuccinic acid is an FDA-approved form of chelation, usually given orally, used in the removal of heavy metals from the body. Consult a medical professional when determining which type of chelation is most appropriate for you.

EDTA Ethylenediaminetetraacetic acid is an FDA-approved form of chelation, often given intravenously, used in the removal of heavy metals from the body. Consult a medical professional when determining which type of chelation is most appropriate for you.

Electro-Dermal Testing
A simple, non-invasive procedure that uses electrodes on the hands and cuticles to determine the presence of a wide variety of toxins in the body.

Essential Oils Typically obtained through distillation, natural oils contain enhanced fragrance and medicinal properties extracted from plant or other source.. Essential oils are used in many cultures to cure a wide range of discomfort and disease.

Frequency Treatments

Treatments designed to measure biological frequencies and emit carefully controlled therapeutic electromagnetic impulses for the purpose of rebuilding organ strength and reducing toxicity. Among the treatments in this category are the Ondamed System, Quint Box and Rife Machine.

Functional Medicine

A medical approach that uses a variety of complementary, integrative, alternative, and conventional diagnostic techniques and therapies to find and treat the cause of malfunctions in the body. Dr. Kessler believes that chronic diseases are caused by an underlying imbalance in the body. The imbalance is usually multicausal; in other words, there are usually many causes responsible for a health disorder. Kessler's work is largely based on the discoveries of James Maxwell and the laws of electrodynamics, which he believes will prove to be the basis of medicine millennia from now.

Healing Codes A self-healing system and form of energy medicine developed by Dr. Alex Loyd while searching for a remedy for chronic depression. We harbor beliefs in our cells that stem from adverse childhood experiences (ACEs) and other trauma and pain throughout our life. Those negative beliefs promote fear, anger, resentment, sadness, low self-esteem, and bitterness. The Healing Codes work to re-balance the energy field, eliminate stress, and reprogram the cellular memories that may shut down our healing systems and produce destructive energy patterns. Some ALS patients have reported curing themselves of the disease at earlier stages than when Joe discovered the Healing Codes.

Healing Stones Also known as crystal healing, this modality identifies gemstones with various properties. Amethyst, for example, is believed by some to be beneficial for the intestines; green aventurine helps the heart; yellow topaz provides mental clarity. Stones and crystals can be re-energized, cleansed, and refreshed by soaking them in water while exposed to intense moonlight. Healers have different ideas about which stones possess which properties, but science may eventually discover a frequency connection as with sound. Meanwhile, any object that amplifies intention can work with the subconscious.

Healing Medallions

Medallions or charms inscribed with spiritual or religious symbols can become the focus of prayer or meditation, activating healing.

Homeopathy

A modern system of symptom remedy based on "like cures like," homeopathy works by administering trace amounts of substances in various dilutions to heal on both physical and emotional levels. Remedies that have been reported to help those with ALS include Arsenicum Album, Curare, Phosphorus, Plumbum metallicum, Sulphur. Consult a homeopathic doctor for more information on which remedies are right for you, and in which doses.

The Journey/Journey Work

A book and therapy introduced by Brandon Bays that aims to release and reprogram cellular memories through meditation and visualization exercises.

Laser Therapy

Low-level laser, or cold laser therapy, delivers light energy to the mitochondria in the skin, which easily absorb the light and convert it into cellular energy thanks to a primitive pathway shared by photosynthetic bacteria. It has been used by massage therapists, plastic surgeons and chiropractors to aid in healing, as well as in wound healing, hair growth, pain control, traumatic brain injury, and many more issues. Laser therapy is currently being researched for treating ALS.

The Lemonade Diet

Also known as the Master Cleanse, this liquid-only diet consists of only three things: a lemonade-like beverage, a salt-water drink, and herbal laxative tea. The Master Cleanse was first created in the 1940s and has become popular again recently. There are many variations of this recipe, but the ingredients are generally the same, calling for freshly squeezed lemon juice, organic maple syrup, cayenne pepper, and water in specific measurements. The recipe and detailed information about the diet can be found in the original book, *The Master Cleanser*, by Stanley Burroughs.

Master Cleanse   (See *Lemonade Diet*)

Meridians   Meridians are energy channels in the body determined by Chinese Medicine. Each organ (Heart, Brain, Liver, etc.) governs its own path of energy that circulates through the body. In Western Medicine, these channels were thought to correspond to the lymphatic system, and have recently been discovered to correspond to fetal development.

MMS   A highly diluted solution of (FDA food use-approved) chlorine dioxide and water, the "Miracle Mineral Solution" has antimicrobial properties and has shown to be an effective cure for malaria. It has anecdotally cured some kinds of cancer for 100 years, and has helped many with other "incurable diseases." However, dosages have not been clinically tested and there are safety concerns.

Mud Packs   Mud and herbal concoctions are sometimes spread over parts of the body, and other times applied to a patch that adheres to one's feet. They are intended to assist the body in detoxification by absorbing toxins through the skin. Quality control with these products is not consistent. Generally, it is best to consult an herbalist.

Negative Ions   Known to promote healing and release stress within the body, negative ions are in abundance in the natural world, particularly in forests, at beaches and most intensely near waterfalls. They are created when a molecule gains a negatively charged electron. In the natural world, negative ions are in abundance, particularly in forests, at the beach and most intensely near waterfalls. They are known to promote healing and release stress within the body.

Neurobiofeedback
Also called neurofeedback, this uses real-time displays of brain activity—most commonly electroencephalography (EEG), to teach self-regulation of brain function. Typically, sensors are

273

placed on the scalp to measure activity, with measurements displayed on a computer using video displays or sound.

Neuro-linguistic Programming

Neuro-linguistic Programming, or NLP, is a healing method that unravels brain connections made by our langage patterns, using eye movements, gestures, and visualization. Although Joe did not pursue NLP directly, it is a component of Journey work and most likely a tool used by both Tom and Tamara.

Olfactory Glial Cells

Cells taken from the Olfactory nerve in the nasal passage, known for their ability to regenerate after damage. Such cells can be cultured and transplanted in order to attach to and replace damaged neurons elsewhere in the body. This treatment is also referred to as OEG or OEC.

Positive Ions In nature, positive ions are commonly formed by high winds, dust, humidity and pollution and are at their highest just before an electrical storm. Also known as positively charged ions, they have been demonstrated to have a negative effect on the immune system, respiratory system, and overall stress level. Positive ions are usually carbon dioxide molecules that have been stripped of an electron. Among the common potent generators of positive ions are automobiles, most electrical appliances, air-conditioning systems, fluorescent lights, and electrical and computer equipment.

Quantum Reflex Analysis

QRA involves the use of kinesiology to identify toxicities and nutrient deficiencies.

Quint System The "Quint Station" or "Quint Box" works with Holopathy, a digital energy medicine system that opens up new perspectives for holistic treatment. Holopathy is based on The Chinese Five Element Theory, which works with energetically interrelated acupuncture points. If one organ fails to function optimally, all the others are also impacted with dysfunction. For more information on the Quint System, visit quintsysteme.com.

Rickettsia   A parasite, most often carried by ticks, known for causing Rocky Mountain spotted fever, typhus, trench fever and other similar conditions.

Sound Therapy   A Frequency Treatment administered by listening to a customized set of programmed tones through headphones, which are determined via computer generated voice analysis. This particular therapy contributed significantly to Joe's detoxing program, specifically with a measurable reduction of heavy metals. (See *Frequency Treatment,* and *Voice Analysis*)

Sonic Access   Meditation recordings using audio technology that delivers simultaneous positive and uplifting messages to the ears, tailored for the different sides of the brain. No subliminal messages are used, so you can hear exactly what's being said. Also known as "Paraliminal" recordings.

Stem Cell Treatment
    The use of regenerative cells to treat or prevent a disease or condition. Bone marrow, skin, nasal passage (olfactory nerve), placenta, and umbilical chord are common sources of these cells. Stem cells created from skin cells, for example, can be converted into motor neurons, the cells affected by ALS.

Toxicity   Environmental toxins can play a major role in neurological disorders like ALS, especially heavy metals such as Mercury. Metal toxicity can be measured by hair, blood, or urine analysis, and can be remedied by chelation and/or frequency treatments like Sound Therapy. Everyday toxins like smoke, drugs, alcohol, viruses, radiation, pesticides and processed foods can be dangerous to anyone with compromised health.

Vitaflex   A form of reflexology that involves the massaging of essential oils into meridian points on one's foot that are linked to the vital organs of the body.

vitOrgan Treatment

Also called vitOrgan dilutions, these are organic homeopathic drug specialties in 2 ml ampoules for injection at specific appropriate acupuncture points. Treatment can also be administered through drops, capsules, and pills. For more information, see vitorgan.de.

Voice Analysis   All matter has a base resonant frequency. Studying the sounds created by living organisms is called BioAcoustics. Voice analysis can provide information about ones current state of health, and is used as a diagnostic procedure for applying Sound Therapy. The procedure involves speaking or singing into a microphone, which records the voice and processes it digitally. (See *Sound Therapy*)

Wei Syndrome   One of several degenerative motor neuron diseases in Chinese Medicine that are often diagnosed as ALS in Western Medicine.

Index

Made in the USA
Middletown, DE
22 February 2017